THE SOCIOLOGY OF HEALTH AND ILLNESS IN IRELAND

edited by

ANNE CLEARY
and
MARGARET P. TREACY

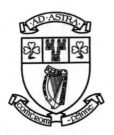

University College Dublin Press
Preas Choláiste Ollscoile Bhaile Átha Cliath

First published 1997 by University College Dublin Press, Newman House, St Stephen's Green, Dublin 2, Ireland

© 1997 The several authors each in respect of the chapter submitted
Introduction © Anne Cleary and Margaret P. Treacy 1997

ISBN 1 900621 11 8

Cataloguing in Publication data available from the British Library

Typeset in Ireland by Seton Music Graphics, Bantry, Co. Cork in 10/12 Ehrhardt
Printed in Ireland by Betaprint

CONTENTS

Introduction

Anne Cleary and Margaret P. Treacy

This book focuses on the contribution of sociology to our understanding of health and illness. The papers included in the collection are diverse in scope and represent, we think, the important contribution that sociology can make to the field of health care. The papers range from theoretical to applied areas but a common feature is their foundation in Irish health issues and society. For the first time, source material concerned specifically with the sociology of health and illness in Ireland is published in one volume. The contributors were each asked to produce a chapter based on recent research or material in their field of specialisation. The papers therefore reflect the main body of original work carried out on sociological aspects of health and illness in Ireland in recent years and as such will inform both the student of sociology and professionals working in the health area.

Health professionals of every kind – all those involved in caring for people in the health services – are becoming increasingly aware of the need to pay attention to more than the disease, to extend their focus beyond what Michel Foucault (1967), refers to as the 'clinical gaze' in order to treat the 'whole person'. This book is therefore aimed at medical, nursing and paramedical students as well as students of sociology, in an effort to bridge the gap between the theoretical aspects of sociology and its applied dimension in health care. This is not a textbook on sociological theory – many books on that already exist – although contributors locate their research within wider theoretical contexts. The main emphasis is on introducing health professionals to sociological work which may inform their practice, and on making students of sociology aware of Irish research in this area. We hope the volume will increase awareness of the relevance and applicability of sociology to health care. The book is organised into four sections and each section deals with the relevance of sociology to various areas of health and health care.

The Sociology of Health and Illness

A sociological perspective on health and illness involves a comprehensive examination of the health area. Broad questions such as the bases and processes of health, illness and disease in society are examined. From the sociological viewpoint the various models or definitions of health are perceived as competing models of health and health care, and the providers and consumers of health are equally important elements in the system. Thus the biomedical or medical model, the dominant definition of health in the western world, is examined alongside alternative approaches to health such as social or holistic models. At a general level, therefore, sociology describes and analyses health, illness and disease and examines how they interact with social, political and economic factors in contemporary society. It is also concerned with the origins and development of health models or definitions of health, as well as with more specific issues such as the experience of health and illness for the individual.

The development of this area of interest reflects trends within and beyond the discipline of sociology in general. Sociology was one of the earliest of the social sciences to study health and illness. Sociology developed in the context of the transition to industrial society, and the large-scale social and population changes which accompanied it. Among the founding fathers of sociology, Auguste Comte (1798–1857) sought to understand the rise of science within that transition, and to establish sociology (a word he invented) on a scientific or 'positive' basis alongside the physical and biological sciences. Karl Marx (1818–83) made lasting contributions to our understanding of the processes which lead from agrarian to capitalist economies, and the dynamics of the social conflicts which accompany them. Max Weber (1864–1920) sought to understand the long-term processes of rationalisation in Western culture, which are manifested in – among many other things – the rise of modern bureaucracies and the 'clinical gaze' itself. All of these theorists continue in their diverse ways to influence the equally diverse work of sociologists today, and some of that influence can be detected in the contributions to this book. But, of all the nineteenth-century figures who formed sociology as the discipline we know today, it was Emile Durkheim (1858–1917) whose work most immediately bore on health and illness. His celebrated study of *Suicide* (Durkheim, 1951), first published in 1897, was one of the earliest investigations of the implications for health and illness of the social changes then in train.

Durkheim's work stands in the 'positivist' tradition, concerned with social structures and how causal factors are implicated in health, illness and disease.

This approach was dominant in the sub-discipline that was then called 'medical sociology' up to the middle of the twentieth century, and it is still important. The work of the American social epidemiologists Faris and Dunham (1939) and Hollingshead and Redlich (1958) exemplify this trend. But other equally important approaches have emerged in recent decades. The origins of the sociological study of illness in the positivist tradition – taking the model of the natural sciences as the ideal – can be seen as closely allied to the medical point of view. Many recent sociologists, however, have consciously stood in opposition to that standpoint. Sociological analysis of the construction of concepts of health and illness, and of the implications of medical discourse and power, have led sociologists on to paths quite distinct from their medical counterparts. This development has been referred to by Strauss (1957) as a move from the study of sociology-in-medicine to the sociology of medicine. The general trend therefore in the sociology of health and illness in recent times has been away from medical definitions and interests to an analysis of the nature and basis of medicine and a shift away from the doctor's to the client's view.

The origins of this change in direction may be traced to work carried out in the last half century. The American sociologist Talcott Parsons (1951), operating within a positivist framework, introduced a number of concepts which were to prove influential in the sub-discipline. In *The Social System* Parsons (1951) underlined the fundamental social nature of sickness and disease. He demonstrated the importance of health to society and how society regulates sickness in order to minimise its disruptive effect. One of the ways this is accomplished, according to Parsons, is through the sick role mechanism. This role provides an exemption from normal role obligations but is conditional on the sick person seeking appropriate, that is medical, help. The sick role therefore legitimises social deviance – behaviour that violates social norms, but is linked to a medical solution or cure. The social control implications of this were later taken up by Scheff (1966, 1975) who, working within a very different theoretical perspective, showed how this process could operate against, and label, certain sections of the population. Goffman's seminal works – firstly on the nature of psychiatric institutions (Goffman, 1961), and later on stigma (Goffman, 1963) continued this examination of the effects of labelling individuals.

Michel Foucault's (1967) writings involve a more general deconstruction of health and medicine than previous theories and are concerned with the development and maintenance of medical discourse and power in society. Central to Foucault's thought is the idea that professional and medical discourses emerged in a particular social, political and historical climate. Thus models of health and healing developed in the context of increased surveillance and regulation in societies, and this extended to the body. He therefore questions the foundations and credibility of medical science – the idea that such knowledge or such a model of health is superior to other models or forms of knowledge. This is in line with postmodernist thinking, which denies the existence of a single theory or explanation for social reality or a unified, linear account of history. The emphasis instead is on multiple realities and histories – on difference and discontinuity. In this view there is a breakdown in knowledge hierarchies, with expert and non-expert having equal status. Thus, within this perspective the patient's experience of illness is equally valid with that of the doctor.

The sociology of health and illness has therefore changed quite significantly in the last forty years, in that it has moved from a position of close association with medicine to a more oppositional stance. There has been a parallel development in theoretical concerns. In the past, medical sociology was, as a number of writers have claimed, theoretically unsophisticated, with conceptual research problems emerging from medicine rather than sociology. The work of writers like Foucault (1967), who has raised issues central to sociology in general as well as to the sociology of health and illness, have changed this. Addressing theoretical issues is now regarded as essential in the contemporary study of health and illness, both to develop specific theory and to link topics to the major theoretical agenda of mainstream sociology. Thus today theorists are operating in a number of areas and at a number of levels, ranging from the experience of illness to wider issues of social structure. The latter include topics such as the role of social constraints in the distribution of health and illness and the social construction of health and disease. The challenge for the sociology of health and illness now, as Turner (1995) has stated, is to link these various theoretical areas and levels together into a cohesive approach. Sociologists in this field are also operating from different viewpoints or paradigms. One contemporary theorist has, somewhat simplistically, divided the main body of workers in the sociology of health and illness into 'structure seekers' and 'meaning seekers' (Pearlin, 1992). Structure seekers in general are concerned with structural concepts in society such as class and family systems and their association with health or ill health. Meaning seekers examine the meaning of social life and its bearing on health and focus on issues such as patients' definitions and experiences of health and illness. The theoretical orientations and methodological foundations of each group therefore vary considerably, with structure seekers tending to use quantitative methods and meaning seekers using qualitative methods. Again this represents a change, as the quantitative approach was the dominant research method in this area up to recent times, reflecting the close association with medicine. However, qualitative approaches have increased in importance and have often proved a more useful and insightful research framework for some topics, such as lay perceptions and attitudes to health. The methodological challenge in the sociology of health and illness may also be to develop a cohesive approach and incorporate both approaches as they are appropriate.

Finally, the area of health and illness has been influenced in recent years by other sociological sub-disciplines, for example gender studies. This latter influence has resulted in a new framework in which to examine the health of both men and women. In particular it has facilitated the emergence of a new, women centred, paradigm in the area of childbirth. The growth of this area of interest is reflected in the present volume with the inclusion of two chapters on aspects of childbirth.

The Changing Nature of Health and Illness

The sociology of health and illness therefore offers a theoretical and applied approach to the study of the health arena. The sub-discipline, as we have noted, has undergone a major shift in orientation and theoretical thinking, due in part to changes within the discipline of sociology itself but also in part to significant shifts in the nature of health, disease and medicine. The nature of health and illness, and with it the whole concept of health and illness, has changed dramatically in the latter part of the twentieth century. In the nineteenth century diseases such as tuberculosis were usually acute and often life threatening. The principal causes of death today are heart disease, cancers, accidents and diseases related to the ageing of the population and changes in lifestyle. The concept of cure, it may be said, has been replaced by concepts of care and rehabilitation. New illnesses such as AIDS have emerged which have profound sociological implications in terms of causation, treatment and prevention. Sociological insight has thus become more important, and there is increasing recognition of the importance of social factors in the occurrence of health problems. There have, in addition, been significant shifts in medicine itself, as the type and nature of disease has changed and there is now increased focus on environmental sources of disease and alternative systems of healing. In the face of this social and health change, established problems, solutions and understandings are challenged because they do not offer adequate solutions. This in turn has led to an erosion of the professional dominance of medicine and the introduction of alternative models or definitions of health and healing. Today the emphasis is more on health than illness and on prevention rather than cure. In terms of prevention there has been an enormous growth of general interest in, and knowledge of, health so that health is no longer viewed as the property of experts. Health, as Nettleton (1995) has said, has become an ubiquitous motif in our culture.

Health and Illness in Irish Society

Ireland as a society has undergone enormous change in the last thirty years. Social, economic and political as well as global factors have contributed to this change. In social terms we have experienced significant changes in marriage and fertility patterns. Substantially more women are now working outside the home and the proportion of single women giving birth and raising children has risen dramatically in the last twenty years. All of these factors have implications for the health system. In health terms our priorities have changed. Our health profile is now in many respects similar to other western countries, but we still retain some rather distinctive health and ill-health features. A principal cause of death in Ireland in mid-century – tuberculosis – is now all but eradicated, and the major causes of death resemble those of other western countries. Cardiovascular disease, in particular heart disease and stroke, is the main cause of death in Ireland (Department of Health, 1995). Suicide, especially among young men, has become a major cause of death and this is in line with figures from other countries (Department of Health, 1996). Yet we have been slow in this country to develop certain health services, particularly in the area of reproductive health for religious and political reasons, and we have shown a tendency to retain institutionalised services (Robins, 1986). There have, however, been significant changes in the health care system in Ireland in the last half century and the health care structure is largely a development of this period. A separate Department of Health was established in 1947 and service expansion developed significantly particularly from the 1960s. In the context of changing health and disease priorities this was a period of scrutiny of existing services. Problems such as tuberculosis were receding and new health priorities relating to population increase and urbanisation were appearing. A particular demographic structure was emerging in Ireland consisting of a high proportion of young as well as older people, and this has had important implications for health and health care. The 1970s saw a move away from institutional treatment and a community care structure was put in place throughout the country. These developments opened up the professional base of health care in Ireland, as the multidisciplinary input into Irish health and health care in effect dates from this period. Thus doctors, who up to this time were the core service providers at least in terms of power and ideological dominance, now in theory began to share this position with other disciplines. In more recent times we have seen the inclusion of research and evaluation as important elements of the health system. Today audit is regarded as essential for evaluating health treatments and processes and more general research is used, albeit less frequently, to assess the experiences and effectiveness of health systems for individuals.

This brief discussion of the direction and origins of sociology and the sociology of health and illness serves as an introduction to the topics of this book of essays. These are the issues and context of this book. More particularly, a sociological lens is useful in examining the health implications of the changing social landscape in Ireland. The complexity and distinctiveness of

Irish society requires specialist examination, and this provided the impetus for the present volume. The essays therefore focus on the contribution of sociology to our understanding of health and illness in the Irish context and offer a framework in which to analyse and reassess existing health issues in Ireland.

Section 1 Sociology, Health and Illness

Section 1 focuses on general and theoretical general issues in the sociology of health and illness. The four chapters included in this section address the relevance of the sociology of health and illness to health care in Ireland, the development of a new health model, lay perceptions of health and illness and the possibilities and dilemmas of technology in medicine. The common theme linking these four papers is that they invite us to stand back and consider some of our assumptions regarding traditional models of health and the promises of new technology. The chapters thus provide a critical and analytical perspective on health care in Ireland.

Sam Porter's paper (Chapter 1) addresses the question of the relevance of sociological insights for health care workers, particularly nurses. Critics of the sociological approach maintain that the concept of individualised patient care is incompatible with sociology and that nursing practice requires a different sort of knowledge. Porter shows how sociology has been used extensively in nursing by nurse educationalists, although the approach has been almost entirely microsociological. This, he claims, has distorted the concept of sociology in nursing and he goes on to argue for the relevance of both macrosociological and microsociological perspectives in nursing practice.

Vincent Tucker's chapter (Chapter 2) critically analyses the bio-medical model of health. According to Tucker this model is built on the assumption that modern medicine has overcome the diseases of the western world. The dominance of the model can be seen in the way in which other health systems are marginalised as 'alternative medicine' or 'non-western medicine'. Tucker argues for a new, more holistic model of health, one that is theoretically precise and is capable of incorporating a variety of therapies including medical treatments. The model Tucker proposes involves two predominant concepts of holism – one focusing on the individual organism and the second on sociological or group dimensions.

In Chapter 3, Desmond McCluskey, on the basis of original research, examines Irish health beliefs and practices. This study showed that health was perceived as multi-faceted by the respondents in that they viewed the physical and mental dimensions of health as equally important. Although health was most frequently conceived of in negative terms, i.e. absence of disease, next in order of frequency came a functional definition – an ability to carry out one's normal roles and tasks. A further, 'reserve' dimension of health was identified in his study – health as a capacity to resist illness. Throughout, perceptions of health were dominated by the bio-medical model, although some change in outlook was indicated.

In Chapter 4, Orla McDonnell examines the social and ethical implications of technology in medicine. She focuses on the social and cultural context which determines how and by whom the technology is used, and refers to a series of contemporary Irish 'case studies' to explore the issues. Although, as McDonnell states, issues concerning the very core of human existence are raised by medical technology, debate on this area in Ireland is conspicuously absent. Thus the cultural assumptions which determine the application of the technology are rarely questioned. Yet the medical profession itself has its own normative assumptions, with which the state appears reluctant to interfere.

Section 2 Inequalities in Health Care

The chapters by Nolan and Whelan and by Collins and Shelley address the topic of social class differences in health in Ireland. Claire Collins's and Emer Shelley's findings (Chapter 5) are based on the Kilkenny Health Project – a longitudinal study of health and illness, particularly coronary heart disease (CHD), in one area of Ireland. The baseline data for this project showed a definite association with social class for various CHD risk factors such as smoking, alcohol consumption, obesity and cholesterol levels. An educational campaign failed in general to improve the relative position of lower social class groupings in relation to risk factors. The findings indicate that education alone is insufficient to lessen class vulnerability, although it is suggested that education campaigns which give due recognition to the cultural context may be more successful.

Brian Nolan and Christopher Whelan (Chapter 6) focus on the relationship between unemployment and ill-health based on various research indicators. Lower socio-economic status is associated with considerably higher mortality rates than for other groups. There is a similar relationship between morbidity and socio-economic grouping, with the percentage of adults reporting long-standing illness at least twice as high for the unskilled manual as for the professional and managerial classes. Further social class differences were found in relation to unemployment and psychological health but people's current employment situation appears to be the more important variable here.

Section 3 Health Issues and Life Course

This section includes a number of essays which demonstrate the application of a sociological perspective and analysis to our understanding of health issues and life-course events. Chapters cover the experiences of pregnant unmarried women, factors underlying teenage pregnancy, caring and the training of carers, and changes in the process of growing older in the last fifty years. All the papers in this section challenge taken-for-granted assumptions regarding the perceptions and needs of client groups. They highlight the need to continue to explore not just clients' perspectives but also the taken-for-granted assumptions of health care professionals.

In a paper based on qualitative data, Abbey Hyde (Chapter 7) describes ways in which childbearing norms can be medicalised. The paper suggests that doctors use moral judgements based on the social circumstances of pregnancy which impact on medical encounters. While the suggestion that moral judgements impact on medical encounters is not entirely new, it is an important phenomenon in the current social context and the climate of client participation in care. It identifies the need to further explore health professionals' own interpretations of such encounters.

In another essay on reproductive health, Finlay *et al.*(Chapter 8) report on a study of teenage pregnancy. They suggest that teenage pregnancy as an issue arose in a context of concern that young unmarried mothers represent a 'burgeoning underclass', with a resultant impact on public spending. This is based on the general assumption that most such pregnancies are unplanned and therefore unwanted. The authors' research explores this assumption and the findings reject a simple dichotomy between planned and unplanned pregnancy. Such categorisation, the study found, fails to capture the complex experiences of how some teenagers came to be pregnant.

In Chapter 9, Orla O'Donovan examines 'caring' with regard to the training of carers of older people. She explores feminist conceptualisations of the concept of caring and the concept employed by statutory health authorities. In reporting on a study which explored views of proposed training for those who care for older people she notes that older people's and family carers' views of caring were different, although both felt that home helps should have some form of training. This is in contrast to statutory health authorities which favour a 'good neighbour' voluntarist approach to such care. O'Donovan suggests that the training debate and arguments against the training of carers are based on gendered assumptions, namely that women do not need training for the 'natural' task of caring, and that such care is not 'real work'. In addition she suggests that it highlights a policy agenda of advocating community care for older people without resourcing this care.

Chapter 10 by Ricca Edmondson again highlights the centrality of the client's perspective in any care-planning activities. She explores the way in which the process of growing older has changed in the last fifty years, particularly in Irish society. She notes that the current emphasis on the growing numbers of older people suggests that they are a static, homogeneous group which, in reality, is not the case. The form growing older takes is heavily dependent on the social setting of the person, and different subgroups have different opportunities and constraints. She suggests that being healthy or well for the older person can only be fully achieved by enabling older people to make their own decisions about public and private processes which impact on them, and by facilitating their integration into society according to their wishes.

Section 4 Mental Health

The focus in this section is on mental health and alcoholism. Tanya M. Cassidy's essay (Chapter 11), based on documentary research, considers the stereotypes which have emerged connecting alcohol and Irishness. This stereotypic view of Irish people as particularly prone to alcoholism has, according to Cassidy, been generally accepted up to recent times. Although the falsity of this view has been known for two centuries, recent work has decisively demonstrated this description of the Irish as alcohol-prone to be amiss. Even so, this myth has influenced many of the conclusions reached by numerous researchers on issues related to alcohol in Ireland.

Anne Cleary's paper (Chapter 12) is an attempt to examine gender differences in relation to mental health data in Ireland. Although information is generally confined to hospital in-patients or out-patients, a picture emerges of a gender differential in terms of diagnosis and positioning within the mental health and hospital landscape. Overall men tend to predominate in the Irish hospital system and this has been the pattern in both the nineteenth and twentieth centuries. Women tend to predominate in the community services. Many of these features are common to mental health systems in other countries, but the excess of male admissions to mental asylums and hospitals in the nineteenth and twentieth centuries appears to be specific to Ireland.

The final contribution by A. Jamie Saris (Chapter 13) examines another crucial element in the history and process of health in Ireland – the asylum. He deals with the evolution of the asylum, setting it in the context of similar developments throughout the world but specifically relating its development to the particular social dynamics of a colonial state. Thus a sterotype emerged, understandable in the colonial context, linking Irishness and insanity yet such a connection was only weakly developed according to Saris. In addressing the present demise of the psychiatric institution system, he again compares the Irish process to the international experience of changing social and medical ways of dealing with the insane.

References

Department of Health (1995) *Health Statistics*. Dublin: Stationery Office.

Department of Health (1996) *National Task Force on Suicide*. Dublin: Stationery Office.

Durkheim, E. (1951) *Suicide: A Study in Sociology*. (Translated by J.A. Spauling and G. Simpson), Glencoe, IL: Free Press.

Faris, R. and H. Dunham (1939*) Mental Disorder in Urban Areas*. Chicago: University of Chicago Press.

Foucault, M. (1967) *Madness and Civilisation: A History of Madness in the Age of Reason*. London: Tavistock.

Goffman, E. (1961) *Asylums: Essays on the Social Situation of Mental Patients and Other Inmates*. Harmondsworth: Penguin.

Goffman, E. (1963) *Stigma*. Englewood Cliffs NJ: Prentice Hall.

Hollingshead, A.B and F.C. Redlich (1958) *Social Class and Mental Illness*. New York, Wiley.

Nettleton, S. (1995) *The Sociology of Health and Illness*. Cambridge: Cambridge University Press.

Parsons, T. (1951) *The Social System*. London, Routledge.

Pearlin, L.I. (1992) Structure and meaning in medical sociology, *Journal of Health and Social Behaviour*, 33: 1–9.

Robins, J. (1986) *Fools and Mad: A History of the Insane in Ireland*. Dublin: Institute of Public Administration.

Scheff, T.J, (1966) *Being Mentally Ill: A Sociological Theory*. New York: Aldine.

Scheff, T.J. ed. (1975) *Labeling Madness*. Englewood Cliffs NJ: Prentice Hall.

Strauss, A. (1957) The nature and status of medical sociology, *American Sociological Review*, 22: 200–4.

Turner, B.S. (1995) *Medical Power and Social Knowledge*. London: Sage.

Section 1

SOCIOLOGY, HEALTH AND ILLNESS

1

Why Should Nurses Bother With Sociology?

Sam Porter

Introduction

This chapter is a bit different from the others in the book. It makes no attempt to address a specific issue of the sociology of health and illness in Ireland. Instead, it takes a step back and discusses whether or not the sociology of health and illness is something that health care practitioners in Ireland or elsewhere should be concerning themselves with at all. However, before getting into this murky debate, it would be useful to say a few words about the reasons as to why sociology has become an integral part of health care knowledge.

The rise of sociology in health care can largely be explained by the gradual demise of what is often termed the 'biomedical' model of health and illness, which saw health and illness as a purely mechanical, physical matter. In its place, a model which spread its explanatory net considerably wider began to emerge:

> It is now realised that the health/illness status is determined not by one factor but many factors . . . Accordingly, it is no longer sufficient to concentrate only on the pathophysiological factors of disease. It is necessary to consider the social factors which contribute to the development of health problems . . .; the cultural factors which determine individual lifestyles . . . ; the environmental factors . . . ; [and] the psychological factors including the manifestation of past experiences in present behaviour (Roper *et al.*, 1985: 4–5).

Thus the claim is that if social factors play a role in the determination of health and illness, then those involved in health care have a responsibility to understand the nature and effects of those factors; hence the need for sociological knowledge.

The sort of knowledge provided by sociology can be divided into two main categories. Firstly, sociological investigations can shed light on the relationship between social situation and patterns of health and illness. Thus, for example, in this book, Anne Cleary examines how gender differences affect the way in which people are likely to use psychiatric services. She points out that, in contrast to Britain, it is men who are more likely to be admitted to psychiatric institutions in Ireland, while women tend to rely more on community psychiatric services. In her examination of how these differentials are related to diagnostic categorisation, Cleary highlights how social factors impinge upon what health professionals might assume to be simply a technical matter of diagnosis.

The second approach adopted by sociologists of health and illness focuses more on health professionals themselves. For example, Vincent Tucker's chapter involves a critique of medical practice as it currently operates, noting that it cannot substantiate its curative claims in practice, and arguing that effective health care requires us to adopt a new health model, namely that of critical holism. The function of this sort of critique is to challenge accepted truths about health care and to provide us with ways of rethinking our attitudes to health and illness.

It may seem obvious that these sort of insights provide very useful information for health care practitioners, showing them how social factors impinge upon health, and how health care might be organised in a more effective manner. Accepting this, we can conclude that practitioners should be aware of these sorts of sociological knowledge. Nevertheless, while all this may sound fairly straightforward, not everyone has been convinced. There has been considerable debate about the merits or otherwise of sociological insights for health care practice. This debate has concentrated specifically on the occupation of nursing, and it is the case of nursing that I will address here. The arguments could, however, be applied equally to other health care professions.

The two major critics of the inclusion of sociology in nursing education have been Hannah Cooke (1993a, 1993b) and Keith Sharp (1994, 1995a, 1995b, 1996). Cooke argues that sociology has been subverted by nursing educators. The reasons for this subversion lie both in vested interests and matters of principle. At the level of interests, she posits that the ambitions of nursing's educational elite have led its members to blunt the critical edge offered by sociology (Cooke, 1993a). At the level of principle, she argues that nursing's belief in the 'individualised care' of patients is incompatible with sociology, in that the unique message of the latter concerns the influence of social structure upon human behaviour (Cooke, 1993b).

More radically, Sharp argues that sociology is an inappropriate form of knowledge for the practical activity of nursing. On the one hand, sociology is so riven by disputes that it is impossible to decide between competing sociological claims, which means that practical health care actions cannot be based with any confidence upon sociological knowledge. On the other hand, sociological ways of thinking, which involve a constant reflection upon and questioning of current knowledge, cannot provide an appropriate framework for nursing thought because nurses require clear and unambiguous knowledge to direct their actions.

These objections raise issues of considerable importance both for health care practitioners and those involved in sociological study. Their importance lies in the questions they raise about the salience of sociological knowledge to the members of the social world which that knowledge describes. Is sociology an irrelevance at best and a danger at worst, or can it provide useful knowledge that can make a benign contribution to the practice of health care? What I propose to do in this chapter is to review these debates and leave you to make up your own mind.

At this point, I have a confession to make. Over the last number of years I have spent quite a bit of time addressing the objections listed above and putting forward arguments to justify the inclusion of sociology in health care education (Porter, 1995, 1996a, 1997; Porter and Ryan, 1996). As a consequence, I can hardly be described as a neutral observer. While I aim to be dispassionate and balanced in my treatment of the various arguments put forward, you should bear in mind where I am coming from as you read the chapter.

Nursing Conservativism

Hannah Cooke's objection to the sociological turn in nursing rests on the contention that nurse educators have undermined the radical message of sociology. Her critique is based upon the philosophy of Michel Foucault, and those social theorists who have applied his work to the contemporary sociology of health and illness. Central to Foucault was his identification of the inseparability of knowledge and power – for Foucault, they were simply two sides to the same coin (Foucault, 1980). In his examination of the rise of modern medicine, Foucault saw the techniques developed by medical science as a form of surveillance which regarded patients as passive objects to be manipulated (1976). While this sort of criticism of the medical approach is familiar enough, Foucauldian critics have applied the same type of critique to holistic care. For them, the inclusion of the social and psychological aspects, in addition to the biological, has the effect of widening the surveillance and power of health care professionals into new areas of the individual's existence. Thus, for example, Armstrong, commenting on nursing's increasing emphasis on communication with patients, states that:

> The nurse is now instructed to communicate with the patient: the patient
> must confess and the nurse must listen . . . From a simple concern with the
> care of the patient's bodily functions, nursing has started to become a sur-
> veillance apparatus which both monitors and evinces the patient's personal
> identity (1983: 459).

Cooke takes up this theme, suggesting that the claims of holistic care to be
empowering to patients, in comparison to more traditional approaches which
reduced patients to their bodily functions and dysfunctions, are without basis:

> The invocation of holism in contemporary nursing contains an explicit criticism
> of . . . techniques of objectification and an appeal to treat the patient as a
> 'whole person'. However holistic nursing heralds not the overthrow of disciplinary
> power but its extension into new realms of individuals' existence (1993a: 213).

Cooke links the increasing adoption of sociology in the nursing curriculum to
the rise of holistic care, observing that the most common justification for
sociology teaching is that it aids understanding of the social and psychological
needs of individual patients. In turn, she associates the rise of holistic care to
the aspirations of 'academic professionalisers' (Melia 1987) within nursing.

Cooke argues that social scientific insights have been incorporated into
nursing knowledge largely on the grounds that if nursing is to be accepted as
a proper profession, it is required to demonstrate possession of a unique body
of scientific knowledge. Sociology is thus being used by academic professionalisers in their attempts to demonstrate that nursing is more than a practical
discipline. It is not hard to see the motivation for this strategy, in that the
status and remuneration afforded to those occupations that are regarded as
true professions are considerably greater than those enjoyed by occupations
regarded as purely practical.

This strategy for professionalisation would be harmless enough if it did not
have profound consequences for the nurse-patient relationship. Here, we see the
influence of Foucault upon Cooke's argument: the theory of sociology is being
used to inform the practice of holistic nursing which in turn involves the surveillance of social and psychological aspects of patients' lives. Cooke thus makes
a three-way linkage in her critique of the application of sociology to nursing:

> It is precisely through the expansion of its surveillance functions that nursing
> lays claim to professional status. And it is as a result of this bid for professional
> status that sociology becomes necessary to nursing (1993a: 214).

She goes on to argue that the implication of this state of affairs is that the
radical aspects of sociology are constrained in the nursing curriculum, in that
they would threaten to uncover the self-serving reasons for which sociology
has been adopted in the first place. Cooke identifies three key ways in which
the message of sociology has been subverted in the nursing curriculum.

Nursing's Subversion of Sociology

Cooke (1993a) argues that sociology has been almost exclusively used by nurse educationalists as a way of understanding the individual. This emphasis tends to limit the perception of social factors to being the property of individuals. Thus, for example, social class is regarded as impinging on health largely through differences in individual attitudes and lifestyles. Lost in such an approach is the idea of class as a form of structured inequality. For Cooke, if nursing ideology is fully accepted,

> the unique message of sociology, i.e. the influence of social structure on human behaviour, must be subordinated to the ideological consensus of . . . [new nursing], which will be concerned with individualized care of patients. Thus the unique message of sociology will be lost (Cooke, 1993b: 1997).

The second, related, constraint involves a lack of emphasis on 'macrosociological' issues – issues concerning large scale social phenomena such as class or gender. Instead, emphasis is almost exclusively on the 'microsociological', which is concerned with immediate, face-to-face interactions. Within nursing curricula, what goes under the name of sociology is often little different from social psychology. Once again, the powerful influence of social structures upon our lives is lost to view.

Finally, Cooke observes that nurses are reluctant to study themselves – either their occupation or the institutions within which they work in a sociological manner. She notes that sociological critiques of the professions and health care institutions get short shrift in nursing curricula, and argues that the reason for this is that such critiques involve unacceptable challenges to current ways of thinking in nursing.

In summary, Cooke's argument is that nurse education has come under the control of academic professionalisers. This elite has an uneasy attitude towards sociology. On the one hand, it is seen as a tool for advancing the professional project, in that it supplies nursing with a body of knowledge. On the other hand, it is regarded as a danger to that project, in that its critical radicalism has the potential to undermine the 'new middle class' pretensions of nursing's educational elite.

Responding to Cooke

Cooke's arguments are both trenchant and acute. What defences can be mounted against them? Let us first address the Foucauldian aspect of Cooke's argument. Acceptance or otherwise of Foucauldian theory rests upon the degree to which one accepts the close connection between knowledge and power. If one accepts that knowledge can be reduced to power then such arguments will seem persuasive. However, the claim that all knowledge can be explained in terms of power is a very large one. As Sahlins (1993) has pointed out, this 'hyper-inflation' of the significance of power ultimately leads to the devaluation of its conceptual currency. Indiscriminate use of the concept of power to explain knowledge can trivialise it as an explanatory tool. As Merquior noted, 'the more you see power everywhere, the less you are able to speak thereof' (1985: 116).

If such critiques of Foucault's perception of power are accepted, then the central objection to Cooke's application of his ideas to nursing would be that while aspirations to power are certainly a factor both in the drive for improved occupational status and the development of new nursing relations with patients, they are not the whole story. Acceptance of the importance of social and psychical factors in the causation and experience of illness, along with the desire to improve communication with patients, while not innocent of self-serving motives, can be interpreted both as providing a deeper under-standing of health and illness (Porter, 1996b), and as promoting the develop-ment of more democratic relations with patients (Porter, 1996c).

Whether we are persuaded by Foucauldian ideas or not, Cooke's more specific accusations about the adoption of sociology by nursing education are well aimed, backed up as they are with evidence from her own experiences of the educational sector. Let us address them in turn.

Nursing's Individualist Sociology

Cooke's assertion that nursing tends to concentrate on the individual to the detriment of social structures seems persuasive. Accepting that there is indeed such a tendency, the only comment that I would like to make is that it can be explained in more traditional sociological terms, without recourse to the extreme scepticism of Foucault (Porter 1996a).

We might observe that, despite state interventions such as the VHI scheme (not to mention church involvement), health care in Ireland, in common with the rest of the Western world, is deeply embedded in the structures of capitalism. This has considerable influence over the sort of care that can be provided. As Navarro (1976) has noted, the interpretation of illness as an individual matter suits capitalism very well, in that it diverts attention away from the socio-economic and environmental causes of illness that result from this form of economic organisation. It could be argued that nursing's individualist approach to sociology reflects this bias. This does not mean, however, that such an approach is inevitable. Indeed, proof of the possibility of a critical nursing approach lies in Cooke's own work, with its exposure of the socio-structural position of nursing.

Nursing's Microsociology

What of Cooke's observation that nursing tends to adopt an exclusively microsociological approach? Once again, I feel we have to accept that there is more than a grain of truth in her argument. However, for at least two reasons, this should not come as a surprise. Firstly, such an emphasis merely reflects a trend in sociology itself. In the 1970s and 1980s, there was a swing away from those approaches which sought to explain the social world in terms of large-scale structures, in favour of approaches which focused on the concrete interactions of individuals. Secondly, it should be remembered that, by and large, nurses care for their patients on a one-to-one basis. Given the micro-social nature of nursing work, it might seem reasonable that nurse education should concentrate on microsociological approaches.

That said, Cooke's observation that nurse education has failed to challenge issues such as inequality, which have a damaging effect on the delivery of care, if true, leaves us with a paradox. On the one hand, understanding individuals' experiences and interactions at a microsociological level is a valid and necessary component of nursing knowledge. On the other hand, exclusive concentration on individual relations blinds nursing to a host of important issues relating to wider institutional and social structures (Porter and Ryan, 1996).

Fortunately, we do not have to make an either/or choice. Since the 1980s especially, one of the prime concerns of social theorists has been to build models that can take account of both social structure and individual action. Probably the most famous of these is Anthony Giddens's (1984) development of structuration theory. The basic premise of structuration theory is that structure and action are two sides of the same coin. On the one side, social structures are created by human actions, and do not exist independently of those actions. On the other side, structures, by providing recognisable patterns, make meaningful interactions between humans possible. The challenge to nursing is to incorporate perspectives such as this, which allow for the significance of social structures without undermining the importance of individual action, into the curriculum.

The Lack of Self-Criticism

Finally, we have Cooke's argument that nurses have been reluctant to study themselves. In response, it has to be said that many of the articles cited in this chapter address this very issue and are to be found in nursing journals. Moreover, the critical analyses in this textbook indicate that it is no longer the case that sociological self-reflection is taboo within health care discourse. This is not to say that we should be complacent; whether or not nursing's use of sociology remains critically reflexive will depend upon nursing academics, educationalists and practitioners being prepared to challenge the assumptions of their occupation.

The Uselessness of Sociology

Cooke's argument is not simply negative; it also prescribes a solution to the problems that she identifies, namely that critical sociological perspectives should be included in nursing discourse. This position has been attacked by Keith Sharp (1995a), who argues that Cooke has misunderstood the practical implications of sociological knowledge:

> sociology is far too diverse and reflexive a discipline to provide straightforward concrete support . . . for Cooke's narrow political vision of what nurse education ought to be about (1995a: 55).

Sharp observes that sociology is not a unified discipline, with a single methodology that all sociologists agree upon. Different sociologists view the world in radically different ways. Moreover, there are no procedures within sociology for settling disputes between different sociologists' approaches. Sharp contends that the problem for nurses about this state of affairs is that different sociological approaches will imply different, and often conflicting, approaches to nursing problems. Because there are no means of deciding which approach is the correct one, nurses are unable to use sociology to guide their actions with any degree of confidence:

> If different sociological hypotheses recommend the performance of different actions in response to practical nursing problems, but sociology can provide no means of ultimately deciding between them, then it seems difficult to avoid the conclusion that sociology is at best worthless to nurses, and at worst, positively harmful (Sharp, 1994: 393).

Sharp further argues that the type of thinking that sociology encourages is not appropriate for the type of thinking that nurses adopt. He notes that sociology is a 'reflexive' discipline – rather than accepting current sociological ideas, sociologists continually reflect upon and challenge that knowledge. In sociology, nothing is certain. By contrast, Sharp argues that nursing work requires an entirely different form of knowledge. Because nursing work is practical, nursing knowledge is concerned with the ways of most efficiently achieving identified goals. Put another way, the sort of knowledge that nurses require is knowledge that can straightforwardly be translated into action. Reflexive sociological knowledge, because it is always unsure of itself, is unable to provide this sort of practical knowledge, and may actually inhibit the ability of nurses to act in a goal-oriented way.

These are strongly stated arguments that may well make nursing readers bridle. However, they are powerfully put and require serious consideration. Essentially, Sharp is making three basic points, which I will engage with in turn. First, he argues that Cooke's call for nursing to adopt a more radical sociological approach is simply a 'narrow political vision'. Second, he contends that, because sociology does not have a unified approach, it cannot guide nurses' actions, because they require more certain knowledge on which to base their actions. Third is his contention that, because sociology is continually questioning itself, it cannot provide the sort of knowledge needed to clearly inform the goal-directed actions of nurses.

Narrow Political Vision

In relation to Sharp's accusation that Cooke's prescription for a radical nursing sociology involves a narrow political vision, it might be argued that whether or not Sharp is correct in his identification of the problems faced by nurses in adopting sociology, Cooke's vision is a widely shared perspective (Porter, 1996a). Readers are directed to Vincent Tucker's chapter on holistic health in this book as an example of how commentators are increasingly asserting the importance of social and environmental factors in the maintenance of health and the production of illness. Critical analysis in relation to health care professions and institutions, along with consideration of wider social factors such as poverty, inequality and industrial organisation, is integral to holistic approaches to care. Cooke's call for a radicalisation of nursing is, then, part of a wider reconsideration of what needs to be addressed if we are to appreciate fully the causation of illness and the requirements of the sick. As such, it is hard to see it as a narrow political vision.

Sociology's Unbridgeable Divisions

Sharp's second argument is that sociology is a deeply divided discipline and therefore of little use to nurses because they are unable to decide which sociological points of view are the correct ones to apply in nursing situations. I think the first thing to note is that he is correct in his observation that sociology is riven by competing theoretical positions. We have already had cause to note, in our discussion of Cooke's ideas, the long-standing division between social structural and social action approaches. Many others could be added to the list – qualitative versus quantitative, Marxist versus Weberian, modernist versus postmodernist, to name but a few. In short, there has never really been a theoretical unity within sociology, nor is there likely to be one in the near future. We therefore have to concede that if nurses do use sociological insights, of whatever hue, they would be very unwise to assume that they have grasped the absolute truth about the social world. However, can we extrapolate from this inevitable uncertainty that sociology can provide no useful information for nursing practice?

My answer to this question has been that such an extrapolation is not warranted because nurses can use various criteria to decide which sociological approaches are most pertinent to their work (Porter, 1995). I identified three criteria which I argued nurses can and do use to decide what sort of knowledge (sociological or otherwise) is appropriate. In order to illustrate my arguments, I used the example of social phenomenology, which is a branch of sociology that examines how people experience and interpret the world, rather than trying to uncover the 'objective' reality of that world.

Pragmatic Utility

The first criterion is termed 'pragmatic utility'. What is meant by this term is that nurses can judge the appropriateness of a sociological position according to its practical usefulness for the job of nursing. Quite simply, those ideas that nurses find most helpful in dealing with the practical day-to-day problems that they face are the ones that they are most likely to adopt.

As we have noted, one of the central aspects of recent developments of nursing has been an expansion away from a narrow concern with the physical signs and symptoms of illness. Nurses now accept that their task is not simply to concentrate on getting people physically better, but also to help them with the wants, needs and fears that arise from the experience of being ill. If nurses are going to be able to do this, they need to know about those wants, needs and fears from the perspective of the people who are feeling them. Thus, social phenomenology, with its emphasis on discovering the experiences, meanings and motives of social actors, will quite clearly be a useful and productive branch of sociology for nurses to know about and apply.

Philosophical Compatibility

The second criterion I identified was 'philosophical compatibility' – the degree to which the philosophy underpinning a sociological perspective is compatible with nursing's own philosophy. Once again, in relation to social phenomenology, it is not simply that nurses might find such an approach practically useful; it is also the case that its philosophical assertion of the crucial importance of subjective experience is highly compatible with the emphasis in nursing philosophy upon the importance of patients' subjective experiences.

Ideological Sympathy

The third and final criterion is that of 'ideological sympathy'. Here, I noted that nursing contained certain values and argued that these values can be used to judge which sociological perspectives are most sympathetic to nursing's concerns. For example, one of the values that is increasingly gaining prominence in nursing is that of feminism. One of the impacts of feminist values upon nursing has been an increasing scepticism about supposedly neutral science, which is regarded as a male-centred form of knowledge, in which the subjects of investigation are reduced to the status of manipulable objects with little say of their own. In contrast, feminist scholars promote a move towards greater valuation of the health-illness experiences of subjects. Thus, the adoption of feminist values leads us once again to a favouring of phenomenological forms of knowledge.

Sharp's Response

Keith Sharp (1996) has subsequently argued that these criteria cannot be used by nurses to decide which sociological theories are best suited to nursing practice. The main thrust of his response is that they are inappropriate because they cannot test the basic truth or falsity of sociological approaches.

> The validity or otherwise of any sociological theory cannot be said to depend upon the point of view of whoever is examining it. Such a move would allow the notion of validity to collapse into incoherent relativism: to say that a statement about the world is true for nurses whilst false for, say, sociologists clearly undermines the very notion of truth, and paves the way for anyone to say anything with equal validity (1996: 1276–7).

According to Sharp, a body of knowledge is either true or false, and this will be so irrespective of whether it is useful for nursing, or if it is compatible with nursing philosophy or values. Accordingly, the criteria I identified cannot be used to decide upon the validity of different sociological claims. As a result, if nurses were to adopt these criteria, they would be in danger of adopting invalid forms of sociological knowledge. For Sharp, knowledge should be judged in terms of truth or falsity, not on its apparent compatibility with the concerns of nurses (or anyone else), be that in terms of practicality, philosophy or value.

The debate has not ended there. My retort to this line of argument has been to contend that it is naive to suppose that any form of knowledge can be judged in the black and white terms of true or false (Porter, 1997). I argue that the idea of being able to discern between absolute truth or falsity has been out of favour with philosophers of knowledge for about the last forty years. It received a serious blow in the 1950s at the hands of Karl Popper (1959) and his principle of falsifiability, which entailed the contention that no matter how many times a theory is tested, it can never be proved to be true. More radically, other philosophers argue that knowledge is the product of the social and historical context in which a producer of knowledge is located, which means that truth can never be seen as an absolute, but something that changes over time and space (for example, Horkheimer and Adorno, 1993[1944]). If such arguments are accepted, then we also have to accept that the best we can do is to use those criteria which we feel are most likely to provide us with the best knowledge possible. That, I argue, is the purpose of the criteria I identified.

Sociology's Reflexivity

Sharp's third objection to applying sociology to nursing is that sociology develops ways of thinking in its students and practitioners that are inappropriate for nurses. The skills involved in sociological thinking, such as scepticism and reflexivity (questioning the grounds of one's own assumptions), because they turn knowledge into a problem, cannot be used by nurses who are required to pursue practical goals.

Sharp is quite correct in his portrayal of sociology as a reflexive discipline, but we need to question whether he is equally correct in his description of nursing as a practical, 'instrumental' discipline (one that uses knowledge simply as a means to get to the practical goals that it has identified). I would argue that this view of nursing is too narrow. Of course it is true that much nursing work is purely practical, requiring instrumental, means-to-ends knowledge. We might think, for example, of setting the rate of an intravenous infusion. If a patient requires a certain amount of a drug to be infused over a certain period of time, then in order to achieve this goal, the nurse will require unambiguous information that will enable her to perform a standard calculation of the number of drips per minute to be infused. However, is nursing work to be confined to this sort of action? We have already talked at length about the new nursing emphasis on more holistic forms of care. One of the basic assumptions of this philosophy is that patients should not be treated as dysfunctional machines – as nothing more than their disease. If nurses were to confine their work to the sort of activity noted above, then that is precisely what they would be doing (Porter, 1996a). Holistic care requires nurses to reflect both on their own activities and on the feelings and understandings of those they are caring for. In other words, nurses require to be reflexive in their work, and would therefore benefit from the ways of thinking adopted in sociology.

Sharp's Response

Sharp's (1996) response to this objection has been to note that the desire of nurses to take into account the patients' perspective and to negotiate rather than impose care plans, though a fine aspiration, is a practical impossibility. He gives two reasons for this. First, he argues that nursing care takes place within bureaucracies, which have a tendency to impose upon those working within them standardised, means-to-end actions. Secondly, the ethos of professionalism to which nursing adheres also produces a standardisation of the ways in which nurses go about their work.

The second of Sharp's reasons is probably the weakest, in that it assumes that nurses view their occupation from a traditional professional perspective. There are good reasons to suppose that, for many nurses, this is not the case.

We have already noted that new nursing does not involve the assumption that, as the professional, the nurse always knows best, and as the client, the patient has nothing of value to contribute to decisions about their care. Instead of this rather old-fashioned view of the professional/client relationship, there has been a general thrust in nursing towards a reworking of that relationship towards a more egalitarian approach (Porter, 1992; Davies, 1995). Thus, it would seem that, at least in terms of the ideas that nurses have about their occupation, it is not the case that there is pressure to standardise nursing work.

While this may be so, it could still be argued that although nurses may wish to work in a non-standardised fashion, in order to allow them to tailor their care to meet the individual needs of patients, the conditions within which they work prevent them from doing so. Here we come to Sharp's first argument that being part of bureaucracy means that nurses have to standardise their work. As any practising nurse will know, the observation that nurses, because of bureaucratic requirements and restraints in resources, are pushed towards task-oriented, rather than person-centred care, has a great deal of truth to it. That is a fact of life with which almost all health care workers have to live.

This dilemma has been identified by Walby *et al.* (1994) in their study of changing professional relationships in the British National Health Service hospital. In contrasting the traditional, standardised organisation of work with more flexible forms of management, they concluded that there was a contradiction between the desire for higher throughput typical of the former, and the patient-centred approach more appropriate to 'new wave', flexible management. They noted that 'the tension between these coexisting logics of management was evident in many issues in the hospital' (1994: 158).

It can be seen that while bureaucracies have traditionally tended towards standardisation, with the developments of new management strategies, such an outcome is not inevitable. Contradictory forms of bureaucratic organisation are competing for dominance within health care systems. Taking this factor into consideration, I would argue that it would be needlessly defeatist of health care workers simply to throw up their hands and accept the inevitability of task-oriented approaches, thus abandoning individualised alternatives. Notwithstanding the difficulties that they will face, nurses and other health care workers do have the option to engage with health care structures and attempt to mould them into a form that is conducive to the performance of individualised care. Ironically, this brings us back to the usefulness of sociology, in that if nurses are serious about implementing new forms of care and are prepared to confront the organisational limits upon the possibility of these forms of care, then surely part of that process will involve the identification and understanding of those structural limits. Where should they go for such understanding? Presumably to organisational sociology.

Summary

The debate between myself and Keith Sharp revolves around how nursing should be conceptualised. First, do nurses require certain knowledge to inform their actions, or can they adopt criteria to decide which sociological insights are more pertinent to their work than others? Second, is nursing a practical occupation, requiring only straightforward, practical knowledge, or does nursing involve social interaction, requiring reflexive knowledge about the nature of interaction? Depending on how these questions are answered, sociology will either be seen as an irrelevance, or as a core part of nursing knowledge.

Conclusion

This paper is a prime example of the sort of self-reflexivity that we have been discussing. It has reflected both upon sociological and nursing knowledge, providing, I hope, a practical demonstration of the compatibility of knowledge styles between the two disciplines. In terms of sociology, the aim has been to encourage sociologists to consider the degree to which their discipline can influence the practicalities of the social world they study, in this case health care. In terms of nursing, the aim has been to allow health care workers to ponder firstly the type of sociology they should adopt, and secondly whether they should adopt it at all. While I have tried to be fair in my account of the debates reviewed here, I do hope that readers have come down on my side of the arguments. This is not just because it's nice to be agreed with. More crucially, if I have ended up, despite my best efforts, leading you to conclude that sociology is of no use to health care professions such as nursing, my name is going to be muck with those who are using this text to teach the importance of sociology. All I ask is that you don't use this chapter as a fine excuse for not doing any more sociological work as a matter of principle.

References

Armstrong, D. (1983) The fabrication of nurse-patient relationships, *Social Science and Medicine*, 17: 457–60.

Cooke, H. (1993a) Why teach sociology? *Nurse Education Today*, 13: 210–16.

Cooke, H. (1993b) Boundary work in the nursing curriculum: the case of sociology. *Journal of Advanced Nursing*, 18: 1990–8.

Davies, C. (1995) *Gender and the Professional Predicament of Nursing*. Buckingham: Open University Press.

Foucault, M. (1976) *The Birth of the Clinic: An Archaeology of Medical Perception*. London: Tavistock.

Foucault, M. (1980) *Power/Knowledge: Selected Interviews and Other Writings 1972–1977*. Brighton: Harvester.

Giddens, A. (1984) *The Constitution of Society*. Cambridge: Polity.
Horkheimer, M. and T. Adorno (1993) *Dialectic of Enlightenment*. New York: Continuum.
Melia, K. (1987) *Learning and Working*. London: Tavistock.
Merquior, J. (1985) *Foucault*. London: Fontana.
Navarro, V. (1976) *Medicine Under Capitalism*. New York: Prodist.
Popper, K. (1959) *The Logic of Scientific Discovery*. London: Hutchinson.
Porter, S. (1992) The poverty of professionalization: a critical review of the occupational advancement of nursing, *Journal of Advanced Nursing*, 17 (6): 720–6.
Porter, S. (1995) Sociology and the nursing curriculum: a defence, *Journal of Advanced Nursing*, 21: 1130–5.
Porter, S. (1996a) Why teach sociology? A contribution to the debate, *Nurse Education Today*, 16 (3): 170–4.
Porter, S. (1996b) Real bodies, real needs: a critique of the application of Foucault's philosophy to nursing, *Social Sciences in Health*, 2 (4): 218–27.
Porter, S. (1996c) Contra-Foucault: soldiers, nurses and power, *Sociology*, 30 (1): 59–78.
Porter, S. (1997) Sociology and the nursing curriculum: a further comment, *Journal of Advanced Nursing*, forthcoming.
Porter, S. and S. Ryan (1996) Breaking the boundaries between nursing and sociology: a critical realist ethnography of the theory-practice gap, *Journal of Advanced Nursing*, 24: 413–20.
Roper, N., W. Logan and A.Tierney (1985) *The Elements of Nursing, 2nd Edition*. Edinburgh: Churchill Livingstone.
Sahlins, M. (1993) *Waiting for Foucault*. Cambridge: Prickly Pear Press.
Sharp, K. (1994) Sociology and the nursing curriculum: a note of caution. *Journal of Advanced Nursing* 20: 391–5.
Sharp, K. (1995a) Why indeed should we teach sociology? A response to Hannah Cooke. *Nurse Education Today*, 15: 52–5.
Sharp, K. (1995b) Sociology in nurse education: help or hindrance? *Nursing Times*, 17(20): 34–5.
Sharp, K. (1996) Sociology and the nursing curriculum: a reply to Sam Porter. *Journal of Advanced Nursing*, 23: 1275–8.
Walby, S., J. Greenwell, L. Mackay and K. Soothill (1994) *Medicine and Nursing: Professions in a Changing Health Service*. London: Sage.

2

From Biomedicine to Holistic Health: Towards a New Health Model

Vincent Tucker

Discussion of health models is usually confined to talking about changes in medical practice, in forms of treatment and diagnosis, or of the addition of some complementary practices such as acupuncture or homeopathy to the medical tool kit. Indeed, much critique of biomedicine[1] remains at the level of criticism of practice or malpractice. But the problem with biomedicine is not that it is ineffective in what it does, but that it is too effective in certain domains to the detriment of other aspects of life and society. It has become a magical fix for all ailments, social as well as physical, and has created an unhealthy reliance on drugs and doctors as well as a questionable use of resources in health care systems. The deeper crisis of biomedicine is summed up by Dr Melvin Konner:

> Doctors and patients alike wait till illness has reached an advanced stage and then look for a quick fix – one that can often cost a fortune and still not work. Almost all of us overestimate what modern medicine can do, and few of us are prepared to face a fact that people in past generations simply could not ignore; all of us must die some time, and if in the process we consume too many of the resources of those who will go on living, we may deny them the kinds of lives we ourselves had (1993: 149).

In sociology, also, most critiques of medicine focus on specific elements of medical practice while not addressing the underlying paradigm.[2] In this chapter I will argue that the limitations of biomedicine are much more deeply rooted than most critiques take into account. They are rooted in a paradigm which has dominated health care and colonised popular imagination since the end of the last decade.

George Engel has argued that the biomedical model has 'become transformed into a folk model, actually the dominant folk model of the Western world. As such it has come to constitute a dogma'. He goes on to argue that dogmas, in contrast to science, maintain their influence through authority and tradition (1980: 543). This folk model is based on a number of myths:

1. The myth that equates health with medicine and the associated belief that the health of a population is dependent on doctors and drugs. In this view doctors are responsible for maintaining the health of a population and the medical expertise necessary for this task is theirs exclusively; and
2. The myth that modern medicine through its discoveries has succeeded in conquering the diseases which ravaged Western societies before the discovery of microbes and modern drugs, that it has increased the longevity of peoples in the Western countries and will eventually do the same for 'underdeveloped' societies.

These myths, despite the fact that they do not stand up to careful scrutiny, have come to be regarded as common-sense knowledge. They continue to be propagated by powerful interest groups such as the medical profession and the transnational pharmaceutical industry. The pharmaceutical industry, which has significantly higher profits than all other industries, spends more than 20% of its earnings promoting drugs but it is also a key promoter of the biomedical approach to health and illness (Tucker, 1996).

It is one of the characteristics of the modern biomedicine that it has hegemonic[3] designs and it has consistently discredited, marginalised or suppressed other systems and practices. The hegemony of biomedicine is reflected in the terms used to refer to other health systems. Notions such as 'alternative medicine' or 'non-western medicine' tend to marginalise other forms of medicine. But despite the fact that biomedicine retains considerable power and prestige it is subject to mounting criticism and its limitations have become more transparent. We are also seeing a proliferation of new approaches to health which include acupuncture, therapeutic massage, homeopathy, yoga, reki, tai-chi. An increasing number of people are beginning to turn to complementary health practices and some biomedical doctors are now practising acupuncture or homeopathy. A recent article in the *Irish Medical Times* argued that 'alternative medicine is a force to be reckoned with'. The article goes on to say that while some biomedical doctors feel threatened and dismiss other medical practitioners as 'charlatans who are merely taking money off people', others see this as a positive outcome and are referring patients to them for the treatment of certain ailments. The Irish Medical Organisation in an advice paper on Indicative Drug Prescribing has recommended that GPs consider sending patients to such therapists as acupuncturists and chiropodists as a cost saving alternative to prescribing drugs.

As we approach the end of the present decade, it is pertinent to ask whether the biomedical paradigm, which has now been in existence for over a hundred years, is on the wane and a new holistic health paradigm emerging. The proliferation of new therapies is not in itself an indication of a paradigm change. Biomedical doctors may use acupuncture in their practice without deviating from the medical model. Moreover, it is important to distinguish between alternative medicines and holistic medicine. Alternative medicines may be holistic, but are not necessarily so. For some practitioners, vitamin therapy or even acupuncture can be used as a cure all in much the same way as antibiotics are used in biomedicine. Holism does not dictate any particular therapy. A holistic practitioner may refer a patient to a biomedical doctor or a hospital clinic for conventional medical treatment and biomedical doctors may recommend therapeutic massage or campaign for cleaner air. Holism is a paradigm which shapes theory and practice and is not reducible to any particular set of therapies. The emergence of a holistic paradigm will require not only a change in the practice of medicine and health care, but also in the knowledge system and the model of science on which it is based. It will also require changes in the institutional fabric of health care.

In this paper I argue that the dominant characteristic of the biomedical paradigm is reductionism, the reduction of a complex set of interrelated factors, social, economic, political, environmental and personal, to one constituent aspect, the biological. It is also reductionist in that it excludes other ways of understanding and practising medicine. I conclude that the limitations of health thinking and practice can only be overcome by the adoption of a more holistic or ecological approach to health. However, the notion of holism is used widely and imprecisely and has come to mean many things to different people. It needs to be theorised more precisely and its practical and methodological implications explored. In this paper I will adopt a sociology of knowledge approach in order to provide a critique of biomedicine, but also to extend the notion of holism beyond its somewhat limited current usage.

The Rise of Reductionist Medicine

I will begin by analysing the process through which the present reductionist model of medicine achieved supremacy over other paradigms. In conventional historical accounts, the emergence of modern biomedicine is portrayed as the achievements of heroes of science such as Pasteur, Koch, Lister, von Behring and Fleming who lifted the veil of obscurantism and discovered the causes of disease which had been hidden for centuries. It is an account of the triumph of science over ignorance and superstition and of the apostles of modern medicine – Schweitzer, Nightingale, Flexner, and others – who brought about a revolution in health care practice and in medical knowledge. The conventional understanding of modern medicine is based on the notion that science provides us with objective knowledge of the true nature of the world. However, all knowledge is necessarily partial and is situated in and reflects particular social and historical circumstances. As Nelly Oudshoorn points out,

> . . . scientific facts do not simply leap into existence as the result of observations by clever scientists who simply read the reality of nature. The myth of scientific heroes discovering the secrets of nature needs to be replaced by another image of science, an image which enables us to study how scientific facts are deeply embedded in society and culture. Not just in the sense that scientific facts shape society, but even the more radical idea that a scientific fact exists only by virtue of its social embeddedness (1994: 10).

In order to understand how knowledge claims – such as the claim of biomedicine that its form of knowledge is superior to other forms of medical knowledge – acquire the status of 'scientific facts', we must examine the processes whereby ideas are promoted, discarded, modified, upheld and accepted to become embedded institutions and practices. Medical facts do not simply emerge when a new technical instrument such as the microscope allows us to uncover previously unknown layers of reality. It took centuries after Van Leeuwenhoek used his microscope to discover that 'animalcules' were present everywhere before this new fact came to be formulated as germ theory.

The construction of 'scientific facts' is not restricted to laboratories somehow hermetically sealed off from the social and political worlds outside them. As the history of the modern pharmaceutical industry demonstrates, laboratory research is in the first instance frequently determined by profit motives rather than by a commitment to the advancement of medical science (Medawar, 1992; Chetley, 1990). The construction of a scientific paradigm, as Thomas Kuhn (1962) has so persuasively argued, has social and political dimensions. The success of scientific ideas goes beyond the laboratory as when scientists build contacts and alliances with other scientists and interest groups who help promote their ideas, and with commercial and political interest groups which provide the economic and political support necessary in order for them to obtain the resources necessary for them to carry out their research. Tales of science are also tales of power.

The rise to hegemony of specific aetiology and its more popular formulation as germ theory illustrates this process. Up until the end of the nineteenth century, most approaches to health and illness were holistic and were based on an environmental and sociological understanding of disease causation and prevention. Hippocrates' treatise 'Airs, Waters, and Places', discussed the relationship between disease and water, soil and winds. Stagnant water and foul air from marshes were believed to cause dysentery, malaria and other ailments. This theory of miasma dominated health thinking and practice until the late nineteenth century. Despite the fact that their knowledge was incomplete, and that the role of amoebas and the anopheles mosquito in the causation of dysentery and malaria were not known, the public health measures to which it gave rise, such as the improvement of water supplies and sanitation, were spectacularly effective in combating these diseases.

A more sociological approach to analysing the patterns and causes of disease epidemics and to taking preventive action emerged in 1662 with John Grant's publication *Natural and Political Observations made upon Bills of Mortality*. This introduced new concepts and the methodology of epidemiology. The bills of mortality which recorded the causes of death allowed for the study of differences in mortality between sexes and between rural and urban populations during the time of great epidemics. The development of advanced statistics by Lambert Quehelet in Belgium, who introduced the notion of age and sex specific rates, the notion of averages, and methods of sampling, further advanced this approach. In France Louis-Rene Villerme developed social biostatistics in 1828 and presented these to the French Academy of Medicine in a memoir comparing death rates of the rich and the poor. This refined epidemiology spread to England where it was used by Edwin Chadwick, a pioneer of the sanitary or public health movement, in his *Report on an Inquiry into the Sanitary Conditions of the Labouring Population in Great Britain* (1842). Chadwick, a disciple of the utilitarian Jeremy Bentham, argued that the root causes of disease were in the poverty and unsanitary conditions of the labouring classes, thus providing a well argued case for social reform as a means of improving the health of the population. Similar arguments were put forward by Sydenham, another pioneer of the sanitary reform movement, who was known as the English Hippocrates. This body of knowledge made a significant contribution to health science and in particular to public health movements. No movement since then has led to such dramatic improvements in public health. This points to the value of sociological insights in understanding disease causation and devising measures to improve health.

Sociological approaches to health were further developed by Friedrich Engels in his first major book *The Conditions of the Working Class in England* (1845) and by Rudolph Virchow in Germany, both of whom emphasised the primacy of social factors in the production of illness. Virchow, who produced more than 2,000 publications in medical science and anthropology, was also an elected member of the German parliament. He is best known today for his research in cellular pathology. His influential *Cellular Pathology* (1860) was the first comprehensive exposition of the basic physiology and pathology of cells. His holistic vision, his multifactorial approach and his emphasis on the centrality of social conditions in the causation of disease were eclipsed by the rise of specific aetiology and are virtually forgotten today. Virchow was an eloquent and influential exponent of the notion that various social, economic, geographic, climatic and physiological factors all play a role in the causation of disease.

He showed how social conditions reducing resistance increased susceptibility to disease. This important insight was eclipsed by the rise of specific aetiology which focused on pathogens as the sole factor in the causation and treatment of disease.

Engels, building on the work of Chadwick, focused on the impact of class structure on health. For him, infectious diseases such as tuberculosis were caused in large part by poor housing conditions. He was aware of the importance of nutrition and discussed the impact of chronic food shortages and high prices. He described rickets as a nutritional problem long before the medical discovery of Vitamin D deficiency. He criticised the inappropriate promotion and misuse of patent medicines and explored the relationship of alcoholism to working conditions. Drawing on the work of Chadwick and others, he carried out epidemiological investigations of mortality and morbidity rates and their relationship to social class. He investigated the relationship between lung diseases and asthma and the working conditions of textile workers, coal miners and metal grinders. His detailed investigations and insights predate later medical findings, but also the contemporary concern with occupational health. He related curvature of the spine, flat feet, varicose veins and leg ulcers to factory work which required long periods of standing.

> . . . all these affections are easily explained by the nature of factory work . . . The operatives . . . must stand the whole time. And one who sits down, say upon a window-ledge or a basket is fined, and this perpetual upright position. This constant mechanical pressure of the upper portions of the body upon spinal column, hips, and legs, inevitably produces the results mentioned. This standing is not required by the work itself . . . (1845: 141–2)

He discussed the problem of lead poisoning, a problem which only re-emerged as a concern in the 1960s and 1970s. From the 1850s onwards, however, these sociological approaches to health were gradually marginalised and replaced by a narrow focus on specific pathogens – the doctrine of specific aetiology.

The shift of attention from social and environmental factors to specific pathogens had more to do with ideology than with biology. There was as yet no scientific basis for germ theory. Major changes in the political climate in Europe followed the reversal of the revolutionary movements and ideas in the period following 1848. The revolution of 1848 gave way to a reaction in the 1850s when the liberal humanitarian impulses which inspired the social reformers gave way to reactionary political ideas such as 'Social Darwinism' which accompanied the rise of capitalism and industrialisation. It became more desirable to hunt germs than to try and find a way to treat social problems. When the new breed of medical practitioners spoke of the 'war against disease' and 'defeating the enemy', they were now referring to invisible enemies such as germs rather than the more visible structures of poverty. The focus on macropathology gave way to a focus on micropathology.

The belief that disease was caused by germs preceded the discoveries of Pasteur and Koch in microbiology by several decades. In 1874, some ten years before these discoveries, F.A.P. Bernard, President of Columbia University, addressed the founding of the American Health Association on the theme of 'Germ Theory and its Relationship to Hygiene'.

> Such has been the success of modern measures for the closing up of all insidious approaches by which disease has hitherto effected its entrance into the family, the community, or the individual organism, as to encourage a hope, even so seemingly wild and visionary, as that a time is coming in which disease itself shall be utterly extirpated, and men shall begin to live out the days which Heaven intended for them (quoted in Gladstone, 1954: 47).

The pre-scientific idea of 'germs' provided what Emily Martin (1994) has referred to as a 'cognitive resource' for the doctrine of specific aetiology. Pasteur was obsessed with germs. He refused to shake hands for fear of contamination. At the dinner table he held glasses up to the light wiping them to remove all contaminating dirt and broke his food into small pieces searching for minute signs of corruption. He was also obsessed with politics, and held extreme right-wing ideas which informed his ideas on germs and which preceded his microbial discoveries. For Pasteur, both germs and the swarming mobs of 1848 were a danger invading and infecting society and he used the same language to describe both (Bodanis, 1995). The laboratory discoveries of Pasteur and Koch were appropriated as scientific proof of germ theory. Germ theory came to capture medical and lay imagination alike. The notion of poverty as the cause of disease was now replaced by the notion of disease as the cause of poverty. Dirt and germs came to be closely associated. Germ theory was further popularised by 'domestic science' texts and the new discipline of home economics, particularly in the USA. These campaigns made both a science and a fetish of cleanliness in the home. At the turn of the century a spate of articles with titles such as 'Books Spread Contagion', 'Infection from Postage Stamps', and 'Germs on Door Knobs' appeared in popular magazines spreading the gospel of germ theory (Ehrenreich and English, 1978). More contemporary manifestations of this legacy include recent articles in Irish newspapers on the dangers of contracting germs from holy water fonts in churches and, in a more commercially motivated vein, the promotion of chemical cleansers which 'kill all known germs'.

The attack on the more sociologically-based understanding of disease causation was led by Emil von Bhering, the man who developed diphtheria antitoxin. Von Behring's *Etiological Therapy* laid the philosophical foundations for the new paradigm of specific aetiology. Because Virchow was the most influential representative of the notion that disease was rooted in social conditions, von Bhering concentrated his attacks on him. Like many contemporary biomedical doctors, von Bhering argued that sociological analyses of the root causes of disease are of little practical value to medicine.

. . . we of this utilitarian age can derive no practical consequences from such a recitation, for palpably Virchow expects little of nothing from medicine and medicaments. For according to Virchow the evil lies too deep to be remedied by mixtures. What is needed, he urged is 'social reform', full and unrestrained democracy. Education with her daughters Freedom and Prosperity (quoted in Galdston, 1954: 52).

However, such arguments were misleading, given the massive improvements made by the sanitary reforms, and in view of the fact that von Bhering's discoveries were still confined to the laboratory (1893). It would be some thirty to forty years before the discoveries of Pasteur and Koch and von Behring would benefit the population at large. Their full impact would await the discovery of sulpha drugs and antibiotics in the 1940s and the emergence of the modern pharmaceutical industry which would cement the final stage of medical reductionism with its promise of a pill for every ill.

It is important to note that opposition to specific aetiology was not based on the idea that microbes played no role in disease causation, but to the claim that they were the sole, entire and singular cause of disease. Virchow and others have sometimes been portrayed as standing in the way of the emergence of the new science but this is unfair and inaccurate. They had no quarrel with the new findings. Indeed, Virchow was a major contributor to modern biomedicine. But, they were opposed to the reductionism which now excluded all other factors as irrelevant. What is significant in this account is the degree to which sociological perspectives were eclipsed by a narrow focus on pathogens. By the end of the century, bacteria had become the central concern of modern medicine and sociological knowledge was marginalised to the point where it was seen as having no place in medical education. biomedicine became a vacuum-sealed domain of expert knowledge whose hegemony continues to be staunchly defended and whose boundaries are jealously guarded against those who argue for the relevance of other forms of knowledge.

The Limitations of Biomedicine

We are only now beginning to emerge from an era in which biomedicine has colonised health knowledge and popular imagination. Its achievements, or perceived achievements, address some of our deepest fears: death, illness, disability. Our relationship to medicine and medical knowledge is not only intellectual, but emotional and moral. Modern culture is replete with stories and legends of great doctors who saved many lives, relieved much pain, and delivered numerous children. They are seen as the self-sacrificing everyday heroes who work hard to protect us and our children from illness and death. Most people have stories of being saved or cured by modern medicine. There are also the public heroes whose spectacular discoveries and achievements inspire awe and hope. Dr Christian Barnard, who performed the first heart transplant, filled the largest soccer stadium in Brazil with crowds of admirers on several consecutive nights; this in a country where most deaths and illness are the result of poverty. The almost magical quality of modern medicines has become part of the everyday lives of peoples everywhere from the Peruvian jungles to the Himalayan mountains. The power of a little white pill to erase pain and fever has become almost legendary. Medical myths are also propagated through soap operas and popular journalism to the point that medicine is akin to a religious belief system. These narratives and icons all play a role in legitimising the myths described at the beginning of this article.

But has biomedicine lived up to its claims? In 1979, Thomas McKeown, in an influential sociological study, *The Role of Medicine: Dream, Mirage, or Nemesis?*, demonstrated that, contrary to widely-held belief, the decline of deaths due to infectious disease so evident at the end of the last century and the beginning of the present century had little to do with medical discoveries such as drugs and vaccines, but resulted from social, political and environmental changes. In 1984, the Minister for Health, Barry Desmond TD, raised probing questions regarding the effectiveness of biomedicine in improving the health of the Irish population.

The argument is often made by critics of our health service that they tend to operate as a self-perpetuating sickness industry rather than as a service designed to ensure maximum health for all. When we look at the indices of contact between the public and the various medical services over the last ten or fifteen years we can see that hospital admissions have been increasing, the number of out-patient consultations has been increasing and the level of activity in General Medical Services has also been increasing. If we look at the figures for the year 1982 we can see that one in every five people in the State was admitted as a new out-patient for consultation and on average each person covered by a medical card had six contacts and was prescribed ten times.

On reflection we must ask ourselves, what is happening to the population that results in these trends. Is the population in some way getting sicker? Or is all this access to the health services making people healthier? We cannot ignore the question whether this commitment of financial and other resources to acute medical services, is achieving a commensurate improvement in the health of the population. Are we, in other words, receiving 'value for effort'. There is some disturbing evidence which suggests that we are not. The life expectancy of Irish people for example is significantly below that of other EEC countries, mainly due to higher death rates among the young and middle aged. Looking at the causes of mortality and morbidity we see that four illnesses and conditions account for 90% of all deaths and for 40% of admissions to acute general hospitals. These are diseases of the circulatory and respiratory systems, cancers and accidents and traumas. Ireland has the dubious distinction of having the highest rate of coronary heart disease in the EEC and the third highest recorded in the world. All of these conditions are closely associated with environment and lifestyle. . . . We must also wonder why, when uniquely among developed countries, the overwhelming majority of the population are in the healthy younger years, we have one of the highest admission rates to hospital of any OECD country. These are just some of the questions which suggest that increased resources in curative care do not seem to be bringing about the benefits of reduced morbidity and mortality which we might expect (Desmond, 1984).

In most industrial countries, the decreasing incidence of infectious disease has not led to an overall reduction in mortality and morbidity, but rather the replacement of one group of illnesses by another group.[4] Stress-related ailments such as ulcers are of epidemic proportions. Millions are spent on drugs such as Tagamet and Zantag to provide relief for sufferers. Cancers, coronary and circulatory ailments, and respiratory illnesses such as asthma, are on the increase. These 'diseases of civilisation' (Inglis, 1983) are due to social and environmental conditions rather than simple biological agents and are not as readily amenable to biomedical treatment as infectious diseases. Indeed, the routine treatment of respiratory ailments with antibiotics is itself contributing to the emergence of iatrogenic illness.

Ivan Illich's trenchant critique in *The Limits of Medicine* (1976) takes the case against biomedicine even further, introducing the notion of medical iatrogenesis i.e illnesses created by medicine.

> Diseases brought on by doctors are a greater cause of increased mortality than traffic accidents and war-related activities. Iatrogenic illness cause between 60,000–140,000 deaths in America alone each year and leave 2–5 million others more or less seriously ill. The situation is worst in establishments which generate medical knowledge, viz. university hospitals where 'one in five patients contracts an iatrogenic disease which usually requires special treatment, and leads to death in one case out of thirty'. With an accident rate like that on his record a military officer would quickly be relieved of his command, a restaurant or a night club would be closed by the police (Illich, 1976).

D'Arcy has produced evidence to show that in the US in the 1980s, over $5 billion a year was spent treating adverse drug reactions. This was close to half the amount spent annually on prescription drugs (D'Arcy, 1986).

Iatrogenic disease is particularly evident in the case of drugs. From its foundations, the modern pharmaceutical industry has brought mixed blessings. It has produced and promoted drugs, such as heroin and cocaine, which have led to massive problems of dependency and addiction (Medawar, 1992; Braithwaite, 1984). The distortions in health care and health spending created by the pharmaceutical industry have now been well documented.[5] The Thalidomide disaster which caused an unknown number of deaths and left at least 8,000 children without legs, arms, ears, and only partially sighted, first awakened the world to the fact that drugs had risks as well as benefits. The SMON (subacute myleo-optic neuropathy) epidemic caused by cloquinol, an ingredient of Mexaform and Entrovioform, brand names for antidiarrhoeal drugs, which left more than 11,000 people (the official figure) paralysed and blind in Japan, revealed an even more sinister picture of pharmaceutical company cover up and intransigence on the part of the medical profession (Hansson, 1989). Medawar, drawing on government and industry sources, has compared injuries requiring hospitalisations and deaths from road accidents and from adverse drug reactions (ARDs). In the UK, road accidents cause around 5,000 fatalities and 60,000 serious injuries each year. Hospitalisations believed to result wholly or largely from drugs amount to 240,000 with 2,500 deaths from ARDs each year (Medawar, 1992: 2–3).

One of the most worrying aspects of modern medicine is that the overuse and abuse of antibiotics, the 'magic bullets' which heralded the end of an era when people routinely died of illnesses such as tuberculosis and pneumonia, is now threatening to take us back to that era. The overuse of antibiotics for prophylaxis, routine and inappropriate prescription for viral infections and minor self-regulating ailments, the production of combination antibiotics, and their use in animal and poultry feed, have all led to significant changes in the internal ecology of the human body. It has led to mass resistance and to the evolution of 'superbugs' such as MRSA (methicilin-resistant staphylococcus) which are difficult or impossible to treat (Cannon, 1995). The seriousness of this epidemic has led the WHO to declare that 'we are standing on the brink of a global crisis in infectious diseases. No country is safe from them. No country can any longer afford to ignore the threat.' From hospital staph infections to candida, new epidemics of antibiotic-related diseases have emerged in recent years. One researcher argues that the increasing incidence of AIDS, cancer, asthma, epilepsy, Alzheimer's disease, rheumatoid arthritis and other difficult to treat diseases is related to the weakening of the human immune system due to the over prescribing of drugs (Vithaulkas, 1991). Yet the reductionist medical paradigm has such a grip on medical knowledge and public culture alike that instead of taking the measures necessary to curb the abuse of antibiotics, health authorities and doctors look towards the pharmaceutical industry to produce new drugs to keep us ahead in the race against mutating bacteria. Despite the seriousness of this threat, and the closure of hospital wards in British hospitals over the past several years, as of the end of 1996 Ireland was the only EU country not to have a national surveillance unit to monitor MRSA. Irish prescribing practice and the organisational structure of Irish medicine is still far removed from the practical measures which are necessary to control the epidemics which are emerging at 'the end of the antibiotic era' (McConkey, 1997: 18).

Critiques of medicine have also emerged from the feminist movement and feminist scholarship. The work of Barbara Ehrenreich and Deirdre English (1978) further extends critical sociological analysis in their feminist history of medicine. Their account of the exclusion of women lay healers from the practice of medicine in the US is especially revealing of the patriarchal basis of biomedicine. The women's movement has also been a rich source of more holistic and self reliant approaches to health care. Publications such as *Our Bodies Ourselves* challenged male medical expertise and provided scores of women with practical health knowledge. Feminists have also carried out extensive research on issues related to reproduction, childbirth, and on drugs for women. Oudshoorn and Coney have shown how research on hormones has further made the female body a site for intervention and manipulation. It has given rise to the establishment of whole new medical industries providing hormones, vitamins, supplements as well as a plethora of medical practices to treat a newly 'discovered' female condition, the menopause (Oudshoorn, 1994; Coney, 1995).

The Emergence of a Holistic Paradigm

Holism is used to describe a heterogeneous family of concepts and practices which have a diversity of origins. While it can be argued that indigenous health thinking and practice is essentially holistic, the systematic articulation of holism as a theoretical paradigm is a more recent phenomenon. It emerged from ecologic theorising in academic circles, particularly in biology, later spreading to the social sciences. Anthropology, and in particular the subfields of medical and ecological anthropology, by virtue of the fact that it straddles the conventional disciplinary divide between biology and the social sciences has made important contributions to the development of new theoretical models.[6] Much of the theorising was underpinned by general systems theory which provided a way of analysing problems from the perspective of wholes rather than parts. The conceptual basis of this approach was developed by Ludwig Von Bertlanffy (1955), a professor of theoretical biology, who was also well versed in psychology and the social sciences. Gestalt psychology, psychotherapy and Buddhist thought have also contributed to the emergence of holism.

In 1959, Rene Dubos, a renowned microbiologist, wrote a series of influential and widely-read books which moved health thinking away from the doctrines of specific aetiology to an ecological view of health as balance between the organism and the environment. In *Man Adapting* (1965), he departed radically from classic microbiology and the notion of malignant germs. He introduced the notion of an internal ecology showing how an imbalance in the indigenous microbial populations could lead to formerly beneficial microbes causing infections which attack the host system. He traced relationships between environmental systems and biological systems linking factors such as nutrition, infection and air pollution. In this view, which challenged popular opinion and medical aspirations, diseases could not be eradicated. Diseases are adaptive systems, and they change in response to alterations in their environment. It is for this reason that eradication strategies, based on the use of insecticides, mass vaccination campaigns, and the mass use of prophylactic drugs can lead to the emergence of resistant strains, whether of mosquitoes or of venereal diseases.

George Engel, a professor of psychiatry, has been one of the main influences in introducing holistic thinking into medical practice. His model, which he calls the biopsychosocial model, uses a systems theory perspective to relate different systems ranging from the cell to society, to the nation, to the biosphere (Engel, 1977). He has translated this theoretical perspective into a form of medical practice which explores a range of possible interventions in addition to conventional interventions such as drugs or surgery. Capra (1989) has developed and popularised holism drawing on concepts and perspectives from anthropology, psychology, biology, and physics, as well as Taoism and Buddhism. Capra recognises the impact of social and economic forces such as agribusiness and chemical companies on health, but his analysis, like most approaches to holism, is less well developed when it comes to incorporating social, economic and cultural systems into the model. Holistic analysis was also influenced by theory and praxis emerging from the environmental movements of the 1970s which were concerned with the destruction of the natural environment and the impact of environmental change and degradation on health. These overlapping concerns and the active, if often strategic, cooperation between environmentalists, feminists, political activists and those concerned with world development gave rise to new syntheses.

Given the wide ranging use of the notion of holism, it might be useful at this stage to distinguish between two versions or tendencies in holistic thinking. One focuses primarily on the individual organism. Most holistic health practice belongs to this tendency. It differs from biomedicine in that in its diagnostic techniques and therapies it takes into account a broader range of systems, which include the biological, the energetic, the psychic, the interpersonal and the spiritual. While it is more cognisant of the social and environmental factors which impact on the health of the individual, and takes these into account in its diagnosis, it does not provide ways of analysing or intervening in these macro systems. The second version of holism derives from the more sociological approach of Engels and Virchow, which predominated before it was eclipsed by specific aetiology. It also derives from the public health tradition. It encompasses economic and political systems as well as biological and environmental systems and is based on the notion that health and illness are not simply biological phenomena but are socially produced. This more sociologically informed holism has been further developed by Marxist political economy and radical development theory (Doyal, 1979; Turshen, 1989). World systems theorists applied the insights and methods of general systems theory to the study of global processes such as the transnational pharmaceutical industry critically examining their impact on health.

To date these two approaches to holism have tended to function somewhat separately from each other, leaving each with its own particular weaknesses. The sociological tradition and radical development theory have focused primarily on the macro-structural dimensions of health and illness. Writers in this tradition have tended to be dismissive of the contribution of holistic therapies because of their emphasis on individual lifestyles and their neglect of macro-level social and political structures. This sociological tradition offers important insights and methodological approaches for the study of the social, political and environmental factors which produce health and illness. It adds a critical edge often missing in holistic health practice. However, it has little to contribute to our understanding of the personal and interpersonal dimensions of illness and well-being. Holistic therapies, on the other hand, provide various means of understanding, exploring and expanding the individual and personal dimensions of human potential usually disregarded by both biomedical and sociological approaches. The critical combination of these two perspectives, which forms the basis of an expanded and more critical notion of holism, can provide a comprehensive alternative to the biomedical model.

Reductionism and Holism: Contrasting Paradigms in Health Care Practice

Reductionism is a methodology which reduces complex wholes to their constituent parts and explains the whole by reference to its smallest parts. Holism, by contrast, refers to 'an understanding of reality in terms of integrated wholes whose properties cannot be reduced to those smaller units' (Capra, 1982: 21). In medicine, reductionist methodology tends to draw attention away from the many different factors – social, economic, environmental, and psychological – which are significant in the production of health and illness and instead gives causal primacy to one particular set of factors, the biological.[7] The focus is on the individual patient and more specifically on the body, which is viewed as a complex machine to be fixed or regulated with drugs or other invasive procedures. Within this system, the more specialised the practitioner the greater their prestige and the more expensive their services. For many consultants, the person and even the body is treated as an appendage to the disease which is their primary concern. This form of medicine is more accurately described as pathology as its concern is with illness and only indirectly with health. It regards social, political and economic factors as outside its remit, focusing only on the proximate causes of disease. As such, it is primarily curative, treating the proximate symptoms which present themselves rather than the root causes of disease.

Biomedical reductionism lends itself to the medicalisation of social problems as when unemployment is treated with valium, air pollution with vasco-dilators, and contaminated water with antibiotics and anti-diarrhoeal drugs. I am not suggesting that ailments such as bronchitis, asthma or amoebic dysentery should not be treated, but that a medical system which restricts itself to treating symptoms while ignoring or claiming to have no responsibility for the conditions which give rise to these is fundamentally flawed. At the level of the individual, the holistic approach is more multi-dimensional, taking into account the energy system, the realm of consciousness, the spiritual dimension, the interpersonal and the social dimension. These concerns are reflected in the therapeutic encounter, in the taking of case histories and in the advice given. In a reductionist approach, other ways of thinking about and treating illness are excluded or dismissed as irrational or unscientific. Alternative medicines also can be reductionist in their methodologies. For some alternative practitioners, vitamin therapy or even acupuncture can be regarded as a cure all in much the same way as antibiotics are used in biomedicine.

From a biomedical perspective, the practitioner is the expert who is responsible for the health of the patient. They take decisions 'in the patient's best interest'. The approach is characterised by paternalism. biomedical practitioners impose diagnosis and treatment and complain about problems of 'non-compliance'. This approach to medicine is based on a professional monopoly of knowledge and responsibility for health. From a holistic perspective, the health practitioner's role is more akin to an educator. The practitioner is a helper who provides expert information and makes the client aware of a range of possible diagnoses relevant to a given health problem or goal. However, the patient assumes responsibility for selecting a diagnosis or treatment regime from among the alternatives presented. This situation approximates self care and the relationship between the practitioner and the health seeker is one of partnership.

From a holistic perspective, most illnesses are regarded as self-limiting and the body, given proper support and a correct environment, can usually heal itself. While medicine may play a part in healing the person or the community, the healing is primarily dependent on corrective action such as changes in lifestyle, in environment, proper nutrition and hygiene. Self reliance does not exclude consulting health practitioners nor the limited and appropriate use of medicines. Neither does it exclude surgical or other medical interventions where appropriate. However, the holistic approach is significantly different from the dominant approach to health care by which practitioners and the public take little or no responsibility for health until a condition becomes chronic and then rely on drugs or other radical interventions. From a holistic perspective, health is not simply a clinically defined state and illness a deviation from that state. Rather, health involves continuing health promoting activity at the individual and the collective level. Reductionist medicine is characterised by a 'pill for every ill' approach to health care. This leads not only to dependence on doctors and drugs, but also leads to entire health systems becoming dependent on the transnational pharmaceutical industry. This 'health industry' has increasingly come to dictate health care practices ranging from forms of diagnosis, to doctor-patient relations, to patterns of treatment, to government spending. Any analysis of government health spending will reveal the extent of this dependence.

A holistic approach recognises that both health and disease are dependent on a variety of interacting factors and that the restoration of health can be achieved in various and often complementary ways. From a holistic perspective, no one group of practitioners or profession enjoys the exclusive right to treat illness. Patients should be free to seek the knowledge and help most appropriate to their health needs. A holistic approach to health promotion, while not excluding biomedical interventions, may include public health practices, environmental campaigns, political action, educational activities and complementary forms of medicine. It will include not only changes in personal lifestyles, but also collective action to challenge organisations and institutions, whether these be tobacco companies, pharmaceutical and chemical companies, or government departments, which act in ways detrimental to public health. From this perspective, campaigns for clean air or food free from antibiotics, hormones and pesticides can play a more significant role in improving community health than increasing the number of cancer specialists, cardiac units or hospital beds.

Conclusion

In the past decade we have seen the emergence of a wide range of new therapies and practitioners in Ireland and elsewhere. A recent survey of 200 people carried out in Cork found that more than 40% had visited an alternative practitioner in the past year. Lay people are becoming more eclectic in their search for treatment, more aware of personal responsibility for their health and more willing to experiment with diet, exercise, meditation, yoga or other such health promoting practices. There is an increasing availability of books, manuals and courses which promote and explain different forms of health knowledge and practice. Acupuncture which was regarded with suspicion in the 1970s and 1980s is now widely established. A growing number of people have at least some familiarity with Chinese, Tibetan or Ayurvedic medicine. There are also an increasing number of professional organisations and practitioners taking a more active role in institutionalising and legitimising complementary health-care systems. Environmental campaigns for cleaner air and unpolluted water are also making an important contribution to the health of the population and generating a more holistic understanding of the causes of illness. There is a growing concern about additives, chemicals, hormones and antibiotics in food and these consumer driven concerns, despite the opposition of powerful vested interests, are coming to be reflected in law. Likewise, groups campaigning against the medicalisation of childbirth, disability action groups, and community-based support groups for various ailments, including psychological ailments, are all contributing towards a less medically centred approach to health and illness. Nursing education is moving towards a more holistic perspective and incorporating perspectives other than biomedicine into its syllabus.

But the monopoly of biomedical knowledge and practice is still firmly established and this hegemony derives considerable support and legitimacy from government funding and legislation. Medical schools remain bastions of reductionist biomedical knowledge and practice and continue to deny the relevance of other perspectives. Medical associations act as institutional protectors of the status quo. Pharmaceutical companies expend a large proportion of their considerable financial resources and political clout in promoting and defending reductionist thinking and practice. Health insurance policies tend to recognise only one form of medical practice as legitimate. In a number of significant ways the institutional dimension of health care lags behind popular practice. This might lead even those who are critical of bio-medicine and see the need for a new approach to conclude that biomedicine is too powerful and too entrenched, both in the institutional realm and in our ways of thinking about health and illness to allow for significant change. This pessimistic view is short-sighted and attributes more coherence and more scientific credibility to the biomedical system than it possesses. In this chapter I have tried to show that the dominance of the biomedical approach to health and illness is a comparatively recent phenomenon historically. In large parts of the world such as India and China, it has never achieved the hegemony which it attained in Western societies. I have also argued that its rise to dominance over other forms of health knowledge and practice has as much to do with political considerations as with its claims to superior scientific knowledge. The establishment of one form of knowledge as superior to other forms depends not only on the coherence of the ideas, but also on the ability of interest groups to promote their claims. This is true in medicine as in other areas of life.

Social systems and knowledge systems do not simply replace one another. Their interactions are much more complex and existing systems are always eclectic. Internal contradictions and inconsistencies do not simply disappear overnight as a health–care system undergoes change. Different dimensions of a system may change at different rates. For example, biomedical practitioners may practise acupuncture without altering their knowledge system. Knowledge systems, practices and organisational systems do not always or even generally shift in tandem. The emergence of a new paradigm involves not only the elaboration of new knowledge, but also a process of social and political struggle to have these knowledge claims recognised. To achieve greater recognition, holistic approaches to health will have to struggle to establish their claims on a number of fronts. One of the weaknesses of the holistic health movement in Ireland has been its failure to articulate comprehensively and persuasively the model on which it is based. This is also an essential prerequisite for entering into dialogue with the established system. Paradigm changes do not come about through revolutionary leaps as Kuhn's analysis suggests, but in a more piecemeal fashion. Changes in practice are not always immediately articulated as a coherent body of knowledge. What we are experiencing in Ireland is a significant shift in health-seeking practices on the part of the general public and some shift in attitudes among biomedical practitioners. These changes have not yet been institutionalised. The purpose of this chapter is to contribute to this change by articulating a critique of the biomedical paradigm which underpins the Irish medical system and by systematically elaborating the philosophical and sociological basis of a more holistic system.

Notes

The Editors gratefully acknowledge the work of Kathy Glavanis in preparing the final version of this chapter following the death of the author.

1   I use the term biomedicine, or biological medicine, to refer to the medical system which predominates in Ireland and in other Western societies. This is usually referred to as the medical model but this usage overlooks the fact that there are a number of medical models including Chinese medicine, Ayurveda, Unnani and Tibetan Medicine. The term allopathic medicine, which means the treatment of disease with drugs having the opposite effects to the symptoms, was coined by Hannemann to describe orthodox medicine as against the system which he founded, homeopathy. It has since entered into widespread use.

2   Stephen Lyng's (1990). *Holistic Health and Bio-Medicine* which focuses centrally on the knowledge systems of each model is a significant exception. In analysing a pardigm we must examine the knowledge system, the practices, and the forms of social organisation. See Tucker, 1995.

3   Hegemony refers to the situation where one form of knowledge and consciousness comes to dominate others in a society. Hegemony operates in two ways: as a form of scientific knowledge advanced by experts and as a form of common sense diffused throughout society.

4   Turshen uses the notion of 'non-specific mortality' to describe the situation where the overall health of a community is not affected by the elimination of any one disease. This is because the particular way in which a society is organised is more important in understanding ill health than clinical or biological information related to specific diseases (1989: 24).

5   See Silverman and Lee, 1974; Melrose, 1982; Medawar, 1984; Chetley, 1990; Tucker, 1990.

6   One of the earliest anthropological contributions was in the study of sickle-cell anaemia where it devised a unitary model for the study of the interrelations between social, environmental and biological factors. The most significant ecological theorist in anthropology was Gregory Bateson (1972, 1979) whose work has influenced several disciplines.

7   It is important to note that economic, sociological and psychological approaches are also frequently reductionist and generally ignore the significance of biological factors in shaping human behaviour and social organisations.

References

Bateson, Gregory (1972) *Steps to an Ecology of Mind*. New York: Bantam.

Bateson, Gregory (1979) *Mind and Nature: A Necessary Unity*. New York: Dutton.

Bodanis, David (1995) Socialism and bacteria, in John Carey (ed.), *The Faber Book of Science*. London. Faber & Faber: 148–60

Braithwith, Robert (1985) *Corporate Crime in the Pharmaceutical Industry*. London: Routledge.

Cannon, Geoffrey (1995) *Superbug: Nature's Revenge. Why Antibiotics Can Breed Disease*. London: Virgin.

Capra, Fritjof (1982) *The Turning Point*. New York: Flamingo.

Capra, Fritjof (1989) *Uncommon Wisdom*. New York: Flamingo.

Chadwick. E. (1965 orig. 1842) *Report on the Sanitary Condition of the Labouring Population of Great Britain*. Edinburgh: Edinburgh University Press.

Chetley, Andrew (1990) *A Healthy Business; World Health and the Pharmaceutical Industry*. London: Zed Press.

Coney, Sandra (1995) *The Menopause Industry*. London: Women's Press.

D'Arcy, P. F. (1986) Epidemiological aspects of iatrogenic disease, in: P.F. D'Arcy and J.P. Griffin, J.P (eds), *Iatrogenic Disease*. Oxford: Oxford University Press.

Desmond, Barry (1984) 'Value for Effort', Address by the Irish Minister for Health to the Health Education Bureau Conference in Athlone, 22 November.

Dobos, Rene (1965) *Man Adapting*. New Haven: Yale University Press.

Dobos, Rene (1959) *Mirage of Health*. New York: Harper & Row.

Doyal, Leslie (1979) *The Political Economy of Health*. Boston: South End Press.

Ehrenrich, Barbara and Deirdre English (1978) *For Her Own Good: 150 Years of Experts Advice to Women*. New York: Doubleday.

Engel, George (1977) The need for a new medical model: a challenge for biomedicine. *Science*, 196: 129.

Engel, George (1980) The clinical application of the biopsychosial model, *American Journal of Psychiatry*, 137: 5

Engels, Friedrich (1973 orig. 1845) *The Condition of the Working Class in England*. Moscow: Progress Publishers.

Galdston, Iago (1954) *The Meaning of Social Medicine*. Cambridge MA: Harvard University Press.

Hansson, Olle (1989) *Inside Ciba-Giegy*. The Hague: ICOU.

Illich, Ivan (1976) *Limits of Medicine: Medical Nemesis: The Exploration of Health*. New York: Boyars.

Inglis, Brian (1983) *The Diseases of Civilization*. London: Granada.

Jewson, N. D. (1976) The disappearance of the sick man, *Sociology*, 10: 225–44.

Konner, Melvin (1993) *The Trouble with Medicine*. London: BBC.

Kuhn, Thomas S. (1962) *The Structure of Scientific Revolutions*. Chicago: University of Chicago Press.

Lyng, Stephen (1990) *Holistic Health and Biomedical Medicine: A Countersystem Analysis*. New York: State University of New York Press.

Martin, Emily (1994) *Flexible Bodies: Tracking Immunity in America from the Days of Polio to the Age of AIDS*. Boston: Beacon Press.

McConkey, Samuel (1997) The end of the antibiotic era, *Irish Medical Times*, 14 (3).

McKeown, Thomas (1976) *The Role of Medicine: Dream, Mirage or Nemesis*. London: Nuffield Foundation.

Medawar, Charles (1984) *The Wrong Kind of Medicine*. London: Social Audit.

Medawar, Charles (1992) *Power and Dependence: Social Audit on the Safety of Medicines*. London: Social Audit.

Melrose, Dianna (1993) *Bitter Pills: Medicines and the Third World Poor*. Cambridge: Oxfam.

Oudshoorn, Nelly (1994) *Beyond the Natural Body: An Archeology of Sexhormones*. London: Routledge.

Silverman, M. and Philip Lee (1974) *Pills, Profits and Politics*. Berkeley: University of California Press.

Tucker, Vincent (1990) Drugs and the distortion of health priorities in developing countries, *Trocaire Development Review*.

Tucker, Vincent (1995) *Critical Holism: Towards A New Health Model*. Cork: Department of Sociology, UCC.

Tucker, Vincent (1996) Health, medicine and development: a field of cultural struggle, *European Journal of Development Research*, 8 (2).

Turshen, Meredeth (1989) *The Politics of Public Health*. London: Zed.

Virchow, Rudolph (1860) *Cellular Pathology*. New York: De Witt.

Vithoulkas, George (1991) *A New Model for Health and Disease*. California: North Atlantic Books.

3

Conceptions of Health and Illness in Ireland

Desmond McCluskey

A major theoretical position in contemporary medical sociology is that of *social constructionism*. According to this view beliefs about health and illness are contingent on their social, cultural and historical context. The same biological phenomena can be interpreted differently in different times and places for social and cultural reasons, and these variations in interpretation can lead to different responses and actions. In other words, definitions of health and illness, perceptions of their causes, and accepted ways of maintaining and restoring health are socially constructed. The dominant paradigm in modern societies for understanding and interpreting health and illness phenomena is what has come to be termed the *biomedical model*: health is viewed simply as the absence of disease, and disease or illness is reduced to a discrete biological abnormality inside the body.[1]

Over the years the biomedical model has been the subject of increasing criticism. The main objections have been outlined by Nettleton: 'The body is isolated from the person, the social and material causes of disease are neglected and the subjective interpretations and meanings of health and illness are deemed irrelevant' (1995: 3). As a consequence of such criticisms, more recent times have witnessed the emergence of an alternative paradigm, the *social model*. This draws attention to the social, economic and environmental causes of health and illness: 'Health is seen as being produced not just by individual biology and medical intervention but by conditions in the wider natural, social, economic and political environment and by individual behaviour in response to that environment' (Jones, 1994: 12). This concern with the complex relationship between people's health and their social and material environment has led to a *holistic* or whole-person approach being viewed as central to health care practice, and as a corollary the patient is to be regarded as an active participant in the therapeutic process, rather than as a passive recipient of medical treatment.

Sociologists, among others, have played a significant role in both the elaboration and promotion of the social model of health. Not only have they time and again demonstrated that health and illness are socially patterned but they have repeatedly affirmed that patients must be treated as whole persons rather than as passive objects. As Nettleton points out: 'Critiques of biomedicine have argued that it is essential to recognise that lay people have their own valid interpretations and accounts of their experiences of health and illness. For treatment and care to be effective these must be readily acknowledged' (Nettleton, 1995: 6). These conceptions or interpretations of health issues constitute collective (social) representations (Durkheim, 1912), in that they are shared by numbers of people and derive from the society or group of which they are members. They refer to commonly held ideas, beliefs and values which inhibit and stimulate action. Central to lay people's representations of health issues are the ways in which they define health and illness and what they perceive as their causes.

Lay Conceptions of Health

Lay health beliefs are those views on health and illness held by ordinary people who are not health professionals. They co-exist with professional definitions and are, to a greater or lesser extent, influenced by them. Up until the 1970s, empirical studies of lay beliefs in Western societies appear to have been very few and confined to the United States, e.g. Apple (1960) and Baumann (1961). With the publication of Herzlich's (1973) pioneering work in France there has been a proliferation of empirical studies, especially in Britain (Blaxter and Paterson, 1982; Pill and Stott, 1982; Blaxter, 1983, 1985, 1987, 1990; Williams, 1983; Cornwell, 1984; Currer, 1986; Calnan, 1987; Stainton-Rogers, 1991; Lambert and Sevak, 1996), but also in France (d'Houtard and Field, 1984, 1986), in the United States (Crawford, 1984), and in the Netherlands (Joosten, 1989). Most of these were small scale studies but those of d'Houtard and Field (1984) and of Blaxter (*Health and Lifestyles*, 1990) were based on very large samples. Although there were variations in the questions addressed and some divergence in the findings the following broad generalisations would appear warranted: (i) definitions of health are multifaceted in that people conceive of health along a number of dimensions; (ii) conceptualisations of health vary among social groups, in particular among social classes; (iii) explanations of health and illness are 'syncretic in origin' (Fitzpatrick, 1984), that is, they are derived from a wide and disparate set of sources; and (iv) lay theories about the causes of health and illness have implications for the actions people take to maintain their health or to remedy illness.

There has been only one published sociological study of the health beliefs and practices of lay people in Ireland (McCluskey, 1989).[2] The objectives of the study were to discover how lay people in general conceive of health and illness and what actions they take to promote 'good' health and to remedy illness. A total of 475 people, randomly selected, were interviewed using a structured questionnaire. Of those interviewed, 47% were normally resident in Dublin city and 53% in a rural community. The present paper is based on the findings of this survey in so far as they relate to the definitions and perceived causes of health and illness of the sample population.

In the survey, the respondents were asked in an open-ended question: 'What do you mean when you say a person is healthy?' Multiple answers were possible. Their replies are shown in Table 1. The results are, in many respects, consistent with those of other studies. Health was found to be a multi-dimensional concept in that approximately two-thirds of the respondents defined health in terms of two or more dimensions or orientations. Health was most frequently conceived of in negative terms, that is, as an *absence of illness*. Next in order of frequency came a *performance* or *functional* definition – an ability to carry out one's normal roles and tasks. Other common descriptions of health were in terms of a *well-being* orientation – one feels good, one is happy and able to cope with life, and a *fitness* orientation – one is physically fit, active, energetic. These results are remarkably similar to those of Blaxter (1987; 1990), and of other studies cited by her: 'Health can be defined negatively, as the absence of illness, functionally, as the ability to cope with everyday activities, or positively, as fitness and well-being' (Blaxter, 1990: 14). With reference to health defined as *absence of illness* McCluskey found, as did Blaxter (1990), that reference to 'disease' was rather rare; when mentioned, it appeared to be used interchangeably with 'illness'.

Table 1 *Definitions of a Healthy Person*

Description	Percentage of Respondents Total Replies*
Illness-free orientation – has no illness	48.8
Performance orientation – is able to work, is able to engage in one's usual activities	33.5
Well-being orientation – feels good, has a good attitude to life	24.0
Fitness orientation – is fit, active, energetic	19.6
Is in good physical and/or mental health	15.2
Other descriptions	30.7
Information incomplete	0.4
N	475

* Percentages sum to more than 100 since more than one answer was possible.

In McCluskey's study a further dimension of health – an *asset* or *reserve* orientation was identified. In reply to the question: 'When two people have no illness is it possible for one of them to be healthier than the other?', 22% of the respondents stated that one person could have a stronger physical constitution or be less susceptible to illness. Thus, health was perceived as a reserve, as a capacity to resist illness. This was one of the principal dimensions of health identified by Herzlich (1973).

It further emerged that almost three-quarters of the respondents in McCluskey's study were of the opinion that health has to do equally with physical and mental well-being. Most of these saw a connection between the two states, that is, mental health influences physical health or vice versa, or that health of mind and health of body go together.

When asked could a person with a serious illness be described as healthy, the vast majority (75%) of the respondents said that such a person could not be so described (Table 2). For most, therefore, absence of *serious* illness was a *sine qua non*, an indispensable condition, for defining a person as healthy.

Table 2 *Health Status of* (a) *Person with Serious Illness*
(b) *A Person with a Serious Physical Disability*

Health Status	Percentage of Respondents	
	(a) Serious Illness	(b) Serious Physical Disability
Could be described as healthy	13.3	62.9
Depends on illness or disability	5.5	2.7
Depends on possibility of cure	4.0	0.2
Other answer	1.6	2.3
Could not be described as healthy	75.6	31.6
Information incomplete	–	0.2
N	475	475

This view runs counter to the findings of Williams (1983) and Blaxter (1990). Williams, in a study of the health beliefs of 70 elderly people in Aberdeen, concluded that it is possible for people 'to refer to someone as healthy even though serious disease is said in the same breath to be present' (Williams, 1983: 189). Blaxter, too, states, in relation to the Health and Lifestyles survey, that 'there are many examples of people who say they are "healthy" despite disease' (Blaxter, 1990: 35). For respondents in Williams's study good health was seen as a reserve, as a power of overcoming disease which is actually present. Blaxter, too, found that people who were suffering from serious conditions were called healthy because they 'coped so well'. She further comments: 'at all ages, but particularly among the elderly, those who themselves were in poor health or suffering from chronic conditions were less likely to define health in terms of illness' (Blaxter, 1990: 21). The results of Williams's and Blaxter's studies suggest that there is less likelihood for the elderly and those with serious illness to define health in terms of absence of illness or disease. This did not emerge from McCluskey's study. The insistence, that a person with a serious illness could not be defined as healthy, was just as common among the elderly and those who had experienced major illness as it was among other respondents.

It is interesting to note that, though most respondents in McCluskey's study were unwilling to ascribe a healthy status to a person with a serious illness, a substantial proportion considered it appropriate to describe a person with a serious physical disability as healthy (Table 2). This is consistent with the respondents' perceptions of the health status of a wheelchair-user who is capable of carrying out normal social roles (see below).

What of less serious illness? It has been observed that nobody experiences perfect health (Twaddle and Hessler, 1977), certainly not in terms of the World Health Organisation's definition as a state of complete physical, mental and social well-being (WHO, 1946). At the same time not everyone is defined as ill – there is a range of less than perfect health within which an individual is still regarded as healthy. McCluskey's findings suggest some of the criteria which lay people employ when they adjudge a person to have moved outside this range and to have entered the area of ill-health. In the first place there is the nature of the symptoms themselves. It emerged that though a person may not be suffering from an illness that is clearly life-threatening, he or she is more likely to be defined as in ill-health when the condition has one or more of the following characteristics: it involves pain (e.g. rheumatism); it is considered potentially serious (e.g. bronchitis); it implies a negative attitude to life; it tends to be chronic, even though mild.

Of major importance was a performance orientation. Persons with non-life-threatening illnesses or conditions who were initially defined as healthy, were very frequently re-defined as being in ill-health when the qualification was added, that because of their illness or condition, they could no longer work or engage in their usual activities. For example, while 89% of respondents would define a man with a heavy cold as basically a healthy person, this percentage is almost halved to 46% when the qualification is added, that because of his cold he is not able to do his work. Again, 74% would regard a man who is a wheelchair-user because of serious leg injuries, but otherwise able to fulfil his usual social roles, as basically healthy; however, only 35% would consider him as healthy when described as unable to work and to do many other things he used to do before receiving his injuries.

There were two dimensions to the performance orientation – an ability to work and an ability to engage in one's usual activities. In the first case there was explicit reference to 'work'; in the second, though work may have been implied it was not specified. Health, defined as an ability to work, was empha-sised most by those in the farming and semi- and unskilled manual occupational groups and least by those in the upper and intermediate non-manual categories; it also tended to receive less emphasis as level of educational attainment rose. Rural respondents more commonly mentioned an illness-free orientation than did those living in the city; the latter more frequently referred to a fitness orientation. As might be expected a fitness orientation received less emphasis with increasing age. Variations in health definitions were unrelated to gender.

When the respondents' perceptions of the relative health status of men and women were examined it emerged that well over half (58%) were of the opinion that men and women are equally healthy. However, a substantial proportion (28% or 133 respondents) considered women to be healthier than men and for the following reasons: women have a stronger constitution and, therefore, are less susceptible to illness; women live longer; they cope better with life; they take better care of their health. In contrast, 66 respondents took the opposite view; men were perceived as healthier than women. The explanations most frequently expressed were: men have a stronger constitution; they exercise more, work harder and are more active; women suffer from more ailments and visit the doctor more frequently. It might be suspected that there would be a gender bias in the respondents' assessments and this indeed was the case. Female respondents were more likely to perceive women as healthier than men while male respondents more frequently defined men as healthier than women. In general, women were perceived as more susceptible to cancer and men more susceptible to heart disease.

Health defined as absence of illness is commonly found in studies of lay health beliefs. In examining health conceptions, the relationship between health and illness invariably arises as it did in the foregoing discussion. Attention will now be directed to the discussion of lay conceptions of illness.

Lay Conceptions of Illness

The respondents' definitions of illness are derived from their replies to the open-ended question: 'What do you mean when you say a person is ill?' Again, of course, multiple replies were possible. The most frequent reply, (43%), was in tautological terms – one is ill when one has an illness (Table 3), though in over a quarter of these the presence of *serious* illness was specified. A substantial proportion of the respondents defined illness in terms of a general performance orientation – one is ill when one is unable to work or engage in one's usual activities (37%). Two other orientations emerged: a medical orientation – one is ill when one requires medical care; and a confinement orientation – one is ill when one is confined to bed or to one's home because of illness.

Table 3 *Respondents' Definitions of an Ill Person*

Definition	Percentage of Respondents Total Replies*
Has an illness/feels unwell	42.5
Is unable to work/Is unable to engage in one's usual activities	37.3
Is confined to bed/house	21.1
Has to attend doctor/in need of hospitalisation	15.4
Other description	10.2
Information incomplete	0.8
N	475

* Percentages sum to more than 100 since more than one answer was possible

Compared with city respondents there was a greater tendency for those in rural areas to describe an ill person as one who needs medical attention or as one who is unable to perform his or her normal social roles including his or her work role. Reference to an inability to perform usual roles increased as educational levels rose.

Cancer and heart disease were identified as the most serious illnesses; one is really ill when one is suffering from these conditions. A large majority of respondents (72%) identified cancer as the most serious of all illnesses. In general, the chances of recovery from the disease were considered poor. Only 17% believed that there is at least a 50/50 chance of recovery; indeed 57% said that there was little or no chance of restoring health. However, the chances of recovery were seen to improve considerably should there be early intervention – in such circumstances 58% considered the chances of recovery to be at least 50/50. People were much more optimistic in their attitudes to heart disease – 44% were of the opinion that, in general, the chances of recovery were at least 50/50 and this increased markedly to 80% should there be early intervention.

The reasons most frequently expressed for regarding an illness as serious were that the condition is incurable or difficult to cure or that it is fatal or usually fatal. Other reasons cited were that the illness leaves one disabled, has serious side-effects, is long-term or that one cannot perform one's usual social roles and becomes dependent on others. These views on the notion of seriousness are strikingly similar to those expressed to Herzlich:

Most frequently seriousness is associated with the danger of dying . . .
Sometimes . . . with the duration or length of the illness . . . The seriousness
of a disorder is also identified with its irreversibility, and with the idea of after
effects or of permanent change of the organism or of the subject's behaviour
(Herzlich, 1973: 67).

Herzlich (1973) has observed that the respondents in her study perceived the
present-day way of life as harmful to the individual and they frequently
referred to different and healthier lifestyles. First there were *references to
the past*. She quotes the remarks of one respondent: 'We always have to be
running, life is more intensively active than before, formerly you lived more
calmly, more healthily'. There were also *references to life in the country*. Life
in the country was seen as natural, healthy and non-constraining, and was
contrasted with urban life which was regarded as imposed upon the human
person. The most important aspects concerned the more relaxed rhythm of
activities and the calmness associated with country life.

In McCluskey's study it was found that, although a majority of respondents expressed the view that those who live on a farm and those who live in
a city are equally susceptible to illness, a substantial proportion (almost two-
fifths) believed that city dwellers are more vulnerable. These views were
unrelated to the respondents' own place of residence. The greater vulnerability
of city dwellers was attributed to the more polluted atmosphere of the city.
Respiratory illnesses, including bronchitis and asthma, were associated with
city life, while brucellosis and other illnesses due to contact with animals
were associated with life on a farm.

Opinion was more divided when respondents were asked to consider the
relative effects on health and illness of life today and life 50 years ago. Over
two-fifths believed that people 50 years ago were less likely to get ill than
people today. That food was uncontaminated and more natural in the past
was the explanation most frequently cited. It was also suggested that there was
less stress, that people were stronger, that they led healthier lives, exercised
more and worked harder. On the other hand, about a quarter of respondents
were of the opinion that people 50 years ago were more susceptible to illness.
This was attributed to two factors: many illnesses are now curable due to
improved medical care, and people today experience a higher standard of living.
The reasons offered here as to why health in general was of a higher or lower
standard in the past are very similar to those expressed to Blaxter (1990)
when respondents were asked why they thought people might or might not
be healthier 'than in their parents' time'.

Perceived Causes of Health and Illness

The respondents' perceptions of the causes of health and illness were derived initially from their answers to three open-ended questions: (i) What would you see as the principal causes of good health in people? (ii) What do you think are the main causes of physical illness? and (iii) Is there anything in the modern way of life that causes illness? In respect of illness causation the focus was on *physical* illness. Again multiple answers were possible. The replies are shown in Tables 4, 5 and 6.

Table 4 *Perceptions of the Principal Causes of Good Health*

Causes	Percentage of Respondents Total Replies*
Good food, healthy food	61.9
Physical exercise, physical hard work, being physically active	37.1
Healthy lifestyle, sufficient rest	26.3
Fresh air	17.7
Being happy, having a positive attitude to life	10.7
No smoking, no drinking, moderation in smoking, moderation in drinking	10.1
Other cause	36.8
Information incomplete	1.5
N	475

*Percentages sum to more than 100 since more than one answer was possible.

Table 5 *Perceptions of the Principal Causes of Physical Illness*

Causes	Percentage of Respondents Total Replies*
Bad diet, lack of nourishment, unhealthy food	38.9
Worry, stress, having a negative attitude to life	19.8
Not enough exercise/work, laziness	17.1
Excessive alcohol, smoking	16.8
Immoderate lifestyle, overwork, not enough rest	15.4
Not having regular medical check-ups	10.1
Other cause	45.3
Other answer	4.6
Information incomplete	8.0
N	475

*Percentages sum to more than 100 since more than one answer was possible.

Table 6 *Features of the Modern Way of Life that Cause Illness*

Feature	Percentage of Respondents Total Replies*
Stress, worry, increased pressure of living, pace of life	34.5
Unhealthy food, due to preservatives, freezing, canning, forced growing of crops, injecting of animals	29.9
Excessive alcohol, smoking, drugs	24.4
Pollution of the environment	19.5
Lack of physical exercise, not enough walking	9.1
Unhealthy lifestyle	4.2
Other features	11.8
No feature in modern way of life that causes illness	7.6
Information incomplete/don't know	5.0
N	475

*Percentages sum to more than 100 since more than one answer was possible.

The factor most frequently identified as the main source of health and illness was the food people eat. Good food, healthy food was perceived as the principal cause of good health (Table 4); bad diet, lack of nourishment, unhealthy food were seen as major sources of physical illness (Table 5). One of the features of modern life most commonly identified as contributing to illness was unhealthy food, unhealthy due to preservatives, freezing, canning, forced growing of crops and 'the injecting of animals' (Table 6).

Next to healthy food, the most frequently perceived determinants of good health were physical exercise and a healthy lifestyle (including sufficient rest). In the causation of physical illness considerable emphasis was placed on the part played by stress and anxiety. Stress was viewed as an outcome of the way of life today; people were healthier in the past because life was less stressful. Other factors seen as conducive to physical illness were lack of exercise, environmental pollution, cigarette smoking and alcohol abuse.

References to food and diet as sources of health or causes of illness are found in other studies including Herzlich (1973), Blaxter (1990) and Lambert and Sevak (1996). The perception of stress as a source of illness is also common to these studies. Further, the reasons volunteered by Blaxter's respondents as to why people were less healthy nowadays are almost identical to those presented in Table 6 referring to sources of illness in modern life, and occur almost in the same order of frequency.

Nettleton (1995), drawing on evidence from Pill and Stott (1982), Blaxter (1983), Cornwell (1984) and Calnan (1987), argues that ideas about disease causation are not the same as ideas about the maintenance of health. Calnan states that while the women in his study had clear recipes about how to maintain health, they did not necessarily feel that they were applicable to disease prevention. The data from Tables 4, 5 and 6 do not appear to endorse this position. Perceptions of the principal causes of health (Table 4) correspond very closely to beliefs about the main sources of illness (Table 5) and to beliefs about the major features of modern life that are conducive to ill-health (Table 6). However, in support of Nettleton's argument, there were noticeable variations of emphasis. For example, there were marked differences in the proportions of respondents identifying good food and physical exercise as principal contributory factors to good health and in the proportions defining these same variables as major sources of illness

It must be noted that the respondents were asked in open-ended questions to identify what they perceived as the *principal* causes of good health and of physical illness. The fact that a specific factor was referred to by only a small percentage of respondents does not mean that it was considered unimportant. For example, in reply to a pre-coded question, two-thirds were of the opinion that cigarette smoking is a serious threat to a smoker's health, whereas, at the same time, a much smaller proportion regarded smoking as one of the principal causes of physical illness.

Finally, physical illness was reported as arising largely from factors external to the human person rather than having its source in individual characteristics such as innate constitution or heredity. Only 2% of the respondents referred to innate constitution and 3% to heredity as among the principal causes of physical illness. Further, in response to a pre-coded question, inborn constitution and heredity were identified as playing an important part in illness causation by only 22% and 25%, respectively, of the respondents.

These views are consistent with the findings of Herzlich's study (1973) where the individual was perceived as essentially healthy, and ill-health was regarded as arising from society and its way of life, a product of technology or human activity. Individual characteristics such as heredity, nature or temperament were seen to play a part in the causation of illness but only to the extent that they indicate a variable capacity for resistance to disease.

Theoretical and Research Implications

The present paper is based on a study of the health beliefs and practices of a sample of Irish people (McCluskey, 1989). Its objective was to analyse the conceptions of health and illness of the members of the sample population – how they define health and illness and what they perceive as their causes. This final section is concerned with the theoretical significance of some of the major findings and their implications for further research. Three issues will be addressed: (1) Changes in definitions of health; (2) Sources of beliefs relating to illness causation; and (3) Health and Self-Concept.

1. Changes in Definitions of Health

As pointed out already, health is not a unitary concept. The results of very many studies clearly demonstrate that people tend to think about health along a number of dimensions. Those most commonly encountered are the four most frequently identified in McCluskey's study: an absence of illness; a performance or functional orientation; a well-being orientation; and a fitness orientation. The above classifications are not precisely defined categories so that some degree of overlap is possible. Blaxter (1990) also makes the point that one may have 'good' health in one respect but 'bad' health in another. But more attention needs to be given to the relative weight attached by people to the various orientations and how these emphases tend to alter over time with changing social circumstances. For the vast majority of respondents in McCluskey's study absence of *serious* illness was clearly perceived as an indispensable condition for defining a person as healthy. It is the author's opinion that this view is probably common to most people. The studies of Williams (1983) and of Blaxter (1990) notwithstanding, it is difficult to conceive how a person with a serious disease, especially if life-threatening, is likely to be defined as healthy by substantial numbers of people. This suggests that health definitions are still dominated by the biomedical approach. Also, the tendency to define more and more problems in medical terms – the medicalisation thesis – is likely to strengthen this position.

However, there are forces making for change. David Tuckett (1976) has observed that the treating of life-threatening disease no longer constitutes a major part of most doctors' work in developed societies. Doctors are now increasingly called upon to treat conditions that prevent individuals from performing self-supporting activities or that in some way interfere with their inner sense of well-being. Accordingly, much of a doctor's time is concerned with helping people to react to and cope with handicaps that a condition may bring about. Hence, as Blaxter observes, if 'illness symptoms are a taken for granted experience, or disease is seen as the norm, then health has to be defined in other ways' (Blaxter, 1990: 21).

Self-help groups of disabled persons, as they strive to project a more positive image, also play a significant role in changing emphases in health definitions. McCluskey's study would suggest that their efforts have met with a fair measure of success in Ireland – over 60% of his respondents would ascribe a healthy status to a person with a serious physical disability.

One of the most important factors influencing the priority given to a holistic approach to health care, is the orientation of a society's medical schools. Formerly, the training of medical students was almost exclusively in terms of a biomedical approach; the concern was with the diagnosis and treatment of disease. However, in more recent times increasing emphasis is being placed on the psycho-social dimensions of the patient – on the person with a disease rather than on the disease in the body. In the Republic of Ireland this emerging emphasis is reflected in the establishment, since the late 1980s, of departments of General Practice in all medical schools where a whole-person approach in the training of students is axiomatic (see Shannon, 1992).

It is not being argued here that absence of serious illness will no longer be regarded by most people as a condition for defining a person as healthy, certainly not in the immediate future; rather that much more emphasis will be placed on other dimensions, especially on the well-being and performance orientations. Therefore, what is being called for here is an increase in systematic studies of how social and cultural changes influence the relative emphases placed on the various dimensions of health definitions.

2. Sources of Beliefs Relating to Illness Causation

Very few of the respondents in McCluskey's study made explicit reference to biological factors as causes of illness; heredity and infection were cited by small numbers, less than 20 in each case. But the influence of biological factors would appear to be implied in references to unhealthy food and environmental pollution found in substantial proportions of the replies. On the other hand, large proportions also pointed to such behavioural causes as lack of physical exercise, smoking and drinking, and an immoderate lifestyle (overwork and insufficient rest). References to biological causes obviously reflect the influence of biomedicine. The frequent mention of behavioural factors would seem consistent with the social model which sees the individual lay person playing an active role in matters of health and illness. At the same time, an emphasis on the adoption of a healthy lifestyle in terms of patterns of consumption and exercise, although going beyond the traditional medical model, is a major element in all health education programmes which are largely directed by health professionals.

However, other patterns of life in Ireland in recent times suggest an alternative influence on lay people's beliefs about illness causation. Ireland, like many other countries, has witnessed a phenomenal growth in the 'fitness industry' – the 'specialist' books and magazines on health matters, the health food shops and the health clubs. Indeed, for some people 'healthism' – the elevation of health to a superordinate value – becomes a major pre-occupation. Nettleton (1995) views this as a prime example of the commercialisation of healthy lifestyles. This accent on a high level of fitness, of course, has probably led to a greater emphasis on a fitness orientation in many people's definitions of health.

Finally, for over a decade now there has been considerable debate about health inequalities: are differences in the health status of different groups of people to be explained largely in terms of structural forces beyond the control of the individual or, conversely, in terms of individual lifestyles? The structural approach focuses on the impact of factors such as poverty, unemployment, the distribution of income, working conditions and pollution. There is considerable evidence to indicate that these factors are the main determinants of health inequalities (Townsend and Davidson, 1982; Davey-Smith *et al.* 1990; Blackburn 1991). Explicit reference to the role of such factors in illness causation was very infrequent in McCluskey's study. Mention was made of lack of nourishment (6%), bad housing (5%) and poverty (2%). Poverty may have been implied in general references to food but one would have expected that factors in the social structure, if regarded as highly important in illness causation, would have been expressed in more explicit terms. Why such an important dimension of the social model of health did not emerge as a prominent feature in respondents' perceptions of the causes of illness is an interesting question for sociological enquiry.

3. Health and Self-Concept

A number of writers have drawn attention to the importance of health status for an individual's self-concept. A valuable review and analysis is provided by Nettleton (1995).

One of the most significant findings of McCluskey's study was the importance of a performance or functional orientation in the health definitions of his respondents. An ability to perform one's usual social roles was a major determinant of their perceptions of the health status of persons with non-serious illness. Persons with non-serious illness, who were initially defined as healthy, were very frequently re-defined as being in ill-health when it was perceived, that because of their condition, they could no longer work or engage in their usual activities. This would appear to have major implications for the identity and self-esteem of sick people, especially for those with chronic illness or disability.

One approach in sociology, symbolic interactionism, has focused considerable attention on the idea of the self. An individual's self-concept or self-image is the set of attitudes, beliefs and opinions the person holds about himself or herself. It has two distinct but related elements, a sense of identity (who I am) and a sense of self-esteem (what I am worth). For symbolic interactionists the perceived attitudes and behaviour of others towards one are crucial to the formation of one's self-concept.

An important dimension of an individual's self-concept is his or her health identity. Like other dimensions of identity, one's picture of one's health is influenced, to a considerable degree, by the response one perceives others to make to one's behaviour. Since, therefore, one is more likely to be perceived as healthy if one is able to perform one's usual social roles, it would seem to be in the interest of one who has experienced illness, to return as soon as possible to former roles, including one's work role. Not only would one be relieved of the social stress and isolation that is associated with removal from one's accustomed interpersonal environment, but also one's sense of identity and sense of self-esteem would be very much enhanced.

But it is in respect of people with serious chronic illness or disability that the relationship between the performance orientation and an individual's self-concept has greatest significance. Although a majority of respondents in McCluskey's study expressed the view that a person with a serious physical disability could be regarded as healthy, it emerged that one is less likely to be so defined, if the disability is associated with an incapacity to engage in everyday social activities including the performance of work roles. It would seem then highly desirable that disabled persons should be given every opportunity to participate as fully as possible in the life of the community, including their having access to gainful employment and educational opportunities. But disabled persons tend to find themselves confronted with social as well as physical barriers to the realisation of such aspirations. This would appear abundantly clear from the 1996 Report of the Commission on the Status of People with Disabilities where the social handicaps imposed on disabled persons in Ireland are set out in some detail.

The respondents' expressed views on the part played by heredity in illness causation are also highly relevant to a discussion of the relationship between health and identity. Less than 3% of the respondents in McCluskey's study mentioned heredity as a principal factor in illness causation and almost three quarters stated that they regarded it as playing a minor role or no role whatsoever.

Why then were respondents inclined to deny or minimise the influence of genetic factors? In the author's view, this response is a form of defence mechanism. It is an attempt by the individual to sustain his or her self-esteem, to preserve an image of oneself as essentially a healthy person. Any suggestion of individual weakness or that 'disease runs in one's family' will be strongly resisted. This would be particularly true in the case of stigmatising or life-threatening illnesses. With so much publicity in recent times on genetic issues, a sociological investigation of the relationship between perceived genetic vulnerability and self-image would appear timely.

Conclusion

This chapter was a review of an empirical study of social conceptions, or, in Durkheimian terms, collective representations of health and illness and their causes. Its objective was to discover how lay people in Ireland conceive of these phenomena. In the final section the data were analysed in relation to three areas of theoretical interest, and what were considered important questions for future sociological enquiry were proposed. It is important to remember that people's representations of their world are not just of academic interest. Their explanations of health and illness influence their behaviour. An analysis of this relationship was also a major focus of the study (McCluskey, 1989) on which this chapter is based but limitations of space did not admit of its discussion. Many more sociological studies, employing a variety of research methods, are required to secure a comprehensive understanding of how lay people in Ireland conceive of matters of health and illness.

Notes

[1] Hart (1985: 531–2), Jones (1994: 12) and Nettleton (1995: 3) provide useful summaries of what they consider to be the model's distinctive features.

[2] The fieldwork for the study was completed in 1981 and a comprehensive report was presented to the Health Education Bureau in 1984. The study referred to here, based on this report, was published by the Stationery Office in 1989.

References

Apple, D. (1960), How laymen define illness, *Journal of Health and Social Behaviour*, 1: 219–25.

Baumann, B. (1961) Diversities in conceptions of health and physical fitness, *Journal of Health and Social Behaviour*, 2: 39–46.

Blackburn, C. (1991) *Poverty and Health: Working with Families*. Milton Keynes: Open University Press.

Blaxter, M. (1983) The cause of disease: women talking, *Social Science and Medicine*, 17: 59–69.

Blaxter, M. (1985) Self-definition of health status and consulting rates in primary care, *Quarterly Journal of Social Affairs*, 1: 131–71.

Blaxter, M. (1987) Evidence on inequality in health from a national survey, *Lancet*, 1: 30–3.

Blaxter, M. (1990) *Health and Lifestyles*. London: Routledge.

Blaxter, M. and L. Paterson (1982) *Mothers and Daughters: A Three Generation Study of Health Attitudes and Behaviour*. London: Heinemann.

Bury, M. (1988) Meanings at risk: the experience of arthritis, in: R. Anderson and M. Bury (eds), *Living with Chronic Illness: the Experience of Patients and their Families*. London: Unwin Hyman.

Calnan, M. (1987) *Health and Illness: The Lay Perspective*. London: Tavistock.

Charmaz, K. (1987) Struggling for a self: identity levels of the chronically ill, in J. A. Roth and P. Conrad (eds), *Research in the Sociology of Health Care*, Vol. 6, *The Experience and Management of Chronic Illness*. Greenwich, Connecticut: JAI Press.

Cornwell, J. (1984) *Hard-Earned Lives: Accounts of Health and Illness from East London*. London: Tavistock.

Crawford, R. (1984) A cultural account of 'health': control, release and the social body, in: J. McKinlay (ed.), *Issues in the Political Economy of Health Care*. London: Tavistock.

Currer, C. (1986) Concepts on well- and ill-being: the case of Pathan mothers in Britain, in: C. Currer and M. Stacey (eds), *Concepts of Health, Illness and Disease: A Comparative Perspective*. Leamington Spa: Berg.

Davey-Smith, G., M. Bartley and D. Blane (1990) The Black Report on socioeconomic inequalities in health ten years on, *British Medical Journal*, 301: 373–7.

Durkheim, E. (1965 orig.1912) *The Elementary Forms of Religious Life*. New York: Free Press.

Fitzpatrick, R. (1984) Lay concepts of illness, in R. Fitzpatrick, J. Hinton, S. Newman, G. Scambler and J. Thompson (eds), *The Experience of Illness*. London: Tavistock.

Goffman, E. (1963) *Stigma: Notes on the Management of Spoiled Identity*. Harmondsworth: Penguin.

Hart, N. (1985) The sociology of health and medicine, in M. Haralambos (ed.), *Sociology: New Directions*. Ormskirk: Causeway.

Herzlich, C. (1973) *Health and Illness.* London: Academic Press.

d'Houtard, A. and M. Field (1984) The image of health: variations in perception by social class in a French population, *Sociology of Health and Illness,* 6 (1): 30–60.

d'Houtard, A. and M. Field (1986) New research on the image of health in C. Currer and M. Stacey (eds) *Concepts of Health, Illness and Disease: A Comparative Perspective.* Leamington Spa: Berg.

Jones, L. (1994) *The Social Context of Health and Health Work.* Basingstoke: Macmillan.

Joosten, L. (1989) The structure of the concept of health in the Dutch population, (Colloque) *INSERM,* 178: 71–84.

Lambert, H. and L. Sevak (1996) Is 'cultural' difference a useful concept?: perceptions of health and sources of ill health among Londoners of South Asian origin, in D. Kelleher and S. Hillier (eds), *Researching Cultural Differences in Health.* London: Routledge.

McCluskey, D. (1989) *Health, People's Beliefs and Practices.* Dublin: Stationery Office.

Nettleton, S. (1995) *The Sociology of Health and Illness.* Cambridge: Polity Press.

Pill, R. and N.C.H. Stott (1982) Concepts of illness causation and responsibility: some preliminary data from a sample of working class mothers, *Social Science and Medicine,* 16: 43–52.

Report of the Commission on the Status of People with Disabilities, *A Strategy for Equality,* (undated but issued in 1996).

Stainton-Rogers, W. (1991) *Explaining Health and Illness: An Exploration of Diversity.* London: Harvester/Wheatsheaf.

Shannon, W. (1992) The place of academic general practice in a medical school, *Irish Journal of Medical Science,* 9: 551–5.

Townsend, P. and N. Davidson (1982) *Inequalities in Health – The Black Report.* Harmondsworth: Penguin.

Tuckett, D. (1976) Introduction in D. Tuckett (ed.), *An Introduction to Medical Sociology.* London: Tavistock.

Twaddle, A.C. and A.M. Hessler (1977) *A Sociology of Health.* St Louis: C.V. Mosby.

World Health Organisation (1946) *Constitution.* Geneva: WHO.

World Health Organisation (1984) *Report of the Working Group on Concepts and Principles of Health Promotion.* Copenhagen: WHO.

Williams, R. (1983) Concepts of health: an analysis of lay logic, *Sociology,* 17: 185–204.

4

Ethical and Social Implications of Technology in Medicine: New Possibilities and New Dilemmas

Orla McDonnell

Introduction

At a time when western society is experiencing a proliferation of scientific medicine, there is growing evidence of public disquiet and social contestation about the encroachment of science and medicine into more and more spheres of social life. In order to understand this apparent ambiguity we need to con-textualise the changing face of scientific medicine and how this is underpinned by cultural shifts. There has been a proliferation of sociological texts which attempt to grapple with this tension. For example, within the field of the sociology of health and illness (and the sociology of the body) Lupton (1994) and Turner (1992 a and b) have developed a cultural model for understanding the paradoxes of society's relationship to scientific medicine and how the scientific episteme (the biomedical system of knowledge) prevails as the dominant discourse[1] in structuring common-sense notions of health, illness and disease. For the social science or medical student the importance of the cultural approach is that it demonstrates how the social significance of scientific medicine is less about the role of medicine in defining health and illness than it is about the construction of the 'normal'. In other words, medicine has a normative function in the construction of meaning about everyday life. We experience medicine manifesting itself as cultural necessity in the way in which it is increasingly aligned with, and assimilated into, the beauty industry. Here we are reminded of cosmetic surgery and the opportunities it affords for reshaping and resculpturing the 'body beautiful'. The popularity of health, fitness, diet and beauty regimes are testament to the increased medicalisation of our bodies. Biomedical technology has reshaped our normative conceptions not just of health, but of medicine itself, and our analytical (philosophical) understanding of the body and life processes. Consider, for example, how scientific advancements in recombinant DNA have altered our conception of the body as a discrete genetic package and the implications this has for diagnostic, preventative and experimental medicine – and how this revolutionises what is normatively understood as 'healthy' and 'normal'.

This is the context in which I will explore the ethical and social implications of technology in medicine. The two empirical cases used, which amplify the need to critically reflect on the 'technological imperative' in contemporary medical practice, are the recent public controversies in Ireland concerning life-sustaining technology, and conceptive technologies or new reproductive technologies (NRT). These cases are chosen because: (*a*) the ethical and social implications of these technologies have been the subject of public deliberations; (*b*) the transformation of the concept of life in the moments of conception and death indicates that what was previously taken for granted as 'sacred' or 'natural' can no longer rely on the tradition of accepted beliefs; and (*c*) when traditional belief systems and common-sense understanding become the object of public discourse and investigation we are forced to encounter the cultural contingency of medicine.

In addressing the social and ethical implications of technology in medicine, it is not the technology *per se* which is under investigation, but the social and cultural context which decides how the technology will be used and by whom. The burgeoning feminist literature on the medicalisation of childbirth shows how technology and its application is never neutral: technology is not a thing or an artefact which acts as an autonomous force. Technology has a symbolic value in promoting medicine as a science and in underpinning the legitimacy of the biomedical model. Feminist research shows how the forceps was not only a technical tool adopted by doctors in the early part of the eighteenth century, but its use was governed by an elaborate set of cultural rules which effectively professionalised obstetrics and at the same time marginalised traditional midwifery. It also changed common conceptions of childbirth as a life process, and women as the knowers of the birth experience were displaced by the male obstetrician as the producer of scientific knowledge and, thus, the definer of the birth experience (Martin, 1993: 54–6). Such conceptual and normative changes encoded a new set of social relations, and these changes have also been marked by conflict and resistance. For example, the 'natural childbirth movement' and the 'home birth movement', which are an attempt to demedicalise childbirth and to reassert the role of the community midwife and the woman as subject and knower, are evidence of the growing disillusionment with and resistance to the medicalisation of birth and the scientisation of women's procreative bodies.

The cases chosen here to highlight contemporary dilemmas about the role of technology in medicine will be approached as an analytical comment on how the public imagination is alerted to such 'crises'. The empirical data is drawn mainly from the public media (television documentaries, radio, and the press), which play a significant role in capturing and structuring our collective imagination. The focus on public media is also important when we consider how medicine and science have been transformed into political relations. The question arises, how do we adjudicate the ethical and social sphere in which traditional and common-sense understandings – everyday lifeworld views – are undermined? While the 'social sphere', i.e. societal issues, seems the natural terrain of the social scientist, how do we interpret ethical issues? The increased rationalisation of modernity has meant that more and more spheres of human activity, which have traditionally been guided by 'moral-practical forms of rationality', are increasingly subjected to 'instrumental rationality' and become subjected to legalistic, economic and administrative rationales (Habermas, 1991: 183, also see Habermas in Outhwaite, 1996). While health care is subjected to these rationales by its very position within the political economy of the welfare state, medical practice is also governed by self-regulatory bodies. It is assumed that medical ethical guidelines not only encode professional prudence, but that they also reflect the cultural ethos of a society. However, when fundamental issues such as death and conception become the subject of conflicting interests, moral absolutes become less significant and ethical guidelines become loose currency.

Analytical Questions

The terminally ill patient who breathes with the aid of a respirator, and who is kept alive by a nasogastric or gastrostomy feeding tube, but has no brain activity such as the seventeen-year-old Hillsborough victim Tony Bland,[2] is a product of advances in medical science. So also is the infertility patient under-going In Vitro Fertilisation (IVF) procedures to conceive a child. She undergoes fertility drug treatment (clomiphene) to increase the number of eggs produced coming up to ovulation and to ensure that the time of ovulation can be scientifically calculated; she then undergoes blood tests, urine tests and pelvic examinations. Once her eggs have reached a stage of maturation she is then administered hormone treatment to release the eggs; the eggs may then be collected by laparoscopy which requires a general anaesthetic or by a procedure called Transvaginal Ultrasound-Directed Oocyte Retrieval (TUDOR). The sperm is produced by masturbation and the eggs and sperm are prepared for fertilisation; if the eggs develop into embryos they are implanted into the woman's uterus by catheter (Kaplan and Tong: 256–65).

These technologies have far-reaching consequences not just for the patients involved, but also for society. They raise moral, ethical, legal and social concerns about the concepts of death and conception. They reorder the boundaries between culture and nature and they raise fundamental philosc · phical questions about biological contingency. They alter the concept of tł ʒ body itself. In the case of the PVS patient – the patient who would die without the technological support of the feeding tube or the respirator – the heart is no long the vital organ which determines being alive or being dead, and in this case brain function determines the moment of death. The reconceptualisation of death (from heart-related criteria to brain-related criteria) has led to a legal quagmire in countries which sought to legalise the new concept of death. Life sustaining technologies (artificial ventilation, artificial feeding and hydration) change conceptual practices in relation to death and the terminally ill patient: they raise the possibility of making death knowable and controllable in a context in which there is little sense of the body as 'nature'. This in turn raises questions about the rights of patients to refuse medical intervention, and in the case of the incompetent patient the issue arises as to who has the right to decide for the patient and on the basis of what principles. The rights of the terminally ill patient become increasingly problematic to adjudicate as the corporeal boundaries between life and death become dependent on the technological advances. Cultural norms are being further pushed out by the intervention of technology, and in the next section I will explore how this manifests itself as interpretative conflicts.

The transgression of the symbolic order between culture and nature is also a dominant theme in the debate on the social and ethical implications of NRT. Since the public pronouncements on the first 'test-tube baby', Louise Browne in Britain in 1978, our common-sense understandings of motherhood in particular have been usurped. For example, the expansive techniques associated with IVF procedures have created the possibility of conceptually dividing motherhood into the genetic mother, the gestational mother and the social mother. The technological possibilities for splitting motherhood not only reorients our conceptualisation of motherhood but also raises social, ethical and legal dilemmas about what constitutes motherhood. When we examine the metaphorical construction of the NRT debate we encounter a new lexicon composed of 'test-tube babies', 'designer babies', 'host mothers', 'baby machines', 'surrogates', 'donors', etc. We are not simply speaking here of a metaphorical shift in language, but the practice of reconceptualising reproductive identity and reproductive relations. Michelle Stanworth (1987), for example, argues that the cultural imagery of the 'test-tube baby' negates the fact that babies do not develop in test tubes, but are nurtured and given birth to by women. Similarly, surrogacy is not a 'substitute' for the 'real mother'. The meaning encoded in the very concept of 'surrogacy' pushes the embodied experience of pregnancy and birth of the contracting mother to the back regions of our imaginations. The medicalised concept of donor implies a lesser status to those who are seen as incidental to the technology; at the same time it is naturalised by the association it conjures up with the donation of blood, organs and tissues. The metaphor of the body as a machine, which is a dominant construct in biomedical conceptions of the body, is inverted by feminist critiques of NRT in the use of the metaphor 'baby machine' or 'mother machine'. These critiques argue that NRT practices dissect, split, commodify and repackage women's bodies, reducing women to mere reproductive vessels (Corea: 1988).

In both the case of life-sustaining technology and NRT the distinctions between health and illness, and between natural and unnatural or artificial, are destabilised, so much so that the boundaries between social norms and scientific possibilities become blurred. The salient analytical question which emerges in the context of public policy is, how should we develop and control medical technologies and to what end? The medical indication for intervention is never based on 'scientific facts' alone, and where normative boundaries are being pushed out, there is always a question mark over the possibility of the means becoming an end in itself.

Case One: Life-sustaining Technology and the Terminally Ill

The public controversy concerning Ireland's first case law on the issue of the treatment of a dying patient not only raised questions of a medico-legal type, but it also raised questions about what is assumed to be socially constituted categories. In other words, the notion that we possess answers to the meaning of life and death in the sense that we understand that nature is the ultimate arbiter of biological contingency, i.e. the inevitability of death. We assume that the definition of death concurs with the prevailing values in our society. The 'right to die' case of the 45 year-old woman who was in a 'near'[3] persistent vegetative state for 23 years arose in the summer of 1995. Prior to this there was no case law on the treatment of the dying patient, and there continues to be no statutory provisions governing the rights of the terminally ill patient. This compares to countries where the definition of death and the rights of patients are subjected to formal legal rules which prescribe medical practice. While the move towards statutory regulation further rationalises and demystifies what is assumed to belong to the sphere of the 'sacred' or 'natural', how this move is interpreted is very much structured by the political economy of health. For example, political mandates may be based on an economic rationality concerning the distribution of scarce health resources[4] or it may be premised on a rights idiom which asserts the issue of bodily integrity. When a fundamental issue such as death becomes subject to conflictual interests the law acts as an arbiter and professional medical ethics become subjected to other forms of rationality. It is in this context that the variable interests (of the patient, her family, the medical profession and the state representing the public good) compete to affect social change, and moral values become manifest in political processes. The case elucidates the loose currency of professional ethics in the face of a conflict of interests about the values which underpin the use of medical technology.

In the absence of case law and statutory guidelines the Irish constitution provides an interpretative framework. Tomkin and Hanafin (1995: 144), however, point out that the interpretations of the 'right to die' are premised on philosophical understanding of the 'right to life'. The tension between what the authors point out as interpreting the 'right to life' as a duty or as an individual choice is in sociological terms a tension between different world views, i.e. between a religious and secular world view. The former position holds that life and death are socially pregiven and governed by natural/divine law, and the secular conception views life and death as socially constituted definitions. Both positions, however, adopt value judgements. The constitutional right to privacy and the derivative right to bodily integrity can be interpreted as a right to refuse medical treatment. Justice Costello interprets the constitution as providing for a legally sanctioned right of the terminally ill patient to refuse life-sustaining technology. This interpretation is premised on the 'right to privacy':

> [T]he dignity and autonomy of the human person as constitutionally predicated require the State to recognise that decisions relating to life and death are, generally speaking, ones which a competent adult should be free to make without outside restraint and that this freedom should be regarded as an aspect of the right to privacy which should be protected as a 'person' right by Article 40.3.1 (Costello: 1986, 35 cited in Tomkin and Hanafin, 1995: 148).

The self determination of the terminally ill patient is more problematic to interpret when the patient is not cognitively able to exercise a choice, for example, the PVS and coma patient, the mentally impaired patient or the minor. The issues at the centre of the High Court Ruling (May 1995) which granted the patient the 'right to die' and the Supreme Court Ruling (July 1995) which upheld this right, not only have implications for how we weight the power of the medical profession and its claim to professional integrity, and the power of state and its interest in preserving life against the interests of the patient, but it raises questions about the definition of death itself.

Case Two: New Reproductive Technology and Infertility

The first potentially controversial fertility technology introduced in Ireland was Artificial Insemination by Donor by the Well Woman Centre in 1982. Intra Fallopian Transfer (GIFT) was introduced in 1986 and In Vitro Fertilisation/Embryo Transfer (IVF/ET) in 1989 (Harrison, 1992). More recently a technique known as Intravenous Cytoplasmic Sperm Injection (ICSI) was introduced by the Rotunda Hospital which houses the Human Assisted Fertility Institute, the main IVF clinic in the state (*The Irish Times*, 25 September, 1995). Like the situation of the terminally ill patient and life-sustaining technologies, there is no legislative framework governing the application of NRT, nor have any medico-legal dilemmas been raised in the courts. The absence of statutory guidelines is peculiar in the context of Northern European countries. For example, in Britain following a public enquiry – the Warnock Commission (published in 1984) – a Voluntary (Interim) Licensing Authority was set up by the Royal College of Obstetricians and Gynaecologists and the British Medical Research Council to regulate NRT practices. Following conflict among clinicians and between the regulatory body and clinicians over clinical practice and research, the Human Fertilisation and Embryology Act was introduced in 1990. This established the terms of reference of a statutory authority to regulate clinical practice and encode the legal status of children born from procedures which involve donor sperm (Price, 1993; Tomkin and Hanafin, 1995: 203).

In Ireland, clinical practice is left to the self-regulatory sphere of the medical profession. The Irish Medical Council's ethical guidelines endorse the guidelines of the Institute of Obstetricians and Gynaecologists, which rule out the use of donor gametes in the practice of IVF and the freezing and storage of embryos (this ban is only specified in relation to embryo research); it also stipulates that all embryos produced by IVF should be replaced in the woman's uterus, and that three embryos are the optimum number to be produced in IVF procedures (Medical Council, 1994: Appendix G, 62–3). The Medical Council qualifies this endorsement by specifying that IVF be limited to married couples. Surrogacy and AID (Artificial Insemination by Donor) are neither prohibited nor regulated by statute and they are not covered by the ethical guidelines of the Medical Council.

Biomedical News: Competing Interpretations

'Right to Die'

Between the late spring and autumn of 1995 there was extensive public coverage of the 'right to die' case. Much of this coverage concerned the actual rulings of the courts and procedural issues. However, what concerns us here is how the public debate which ensued was constructed. This is an important aspect to explore given the implications of the ruling for other PVS and terminally ill patients, and as a way of understanding how issues of medical technology and scientific knowledge are bound up with the politics of interpretation. In other words, how the definitions of death and corporeality are publicly contested, and what this tells us about the symbolic status of life-sustaining technology. For example, does death have intrinsic values of its own? Can it be understood and experienced other than as a rationally calculable object of medical technology and knowledge? The political lexicon of the debate reflected the contestation between two competing world views. This is captured by the tension between the argument for self-determination premised on the social and ethical principle of 'quality of life' and the argument that the ruling sanctioned active euthanasia. The competing definitions of death and corporeality raised questions about what causes death: is the cause of death the original pathology, which in the case of the PVS patient was reportedly global irreversible brain damage, or the withdrawal of the life-sustaining technology? This in turn raised questions about the technology and the justification for its application. For example, a nasogastric feeding tube, through which the patient was reported to have been fed for twenty years, may be considered a 'low' technology in the sense that it requires minimum medical management and few risks for the patient. On the other hand, the use of a gastrostomy tube through which the patient was reported to have been fed for the last three years of her life may be considered a 'high' technology in that it requires a general anaesthetic and hence more risks for the patient and a higher degree of medical intervention.

The 'low' and 'high' distinction is not, however, simply premised on technical definitions relating to scientific calculations; it also encodes a normative definition of the patient and the type of care which justifies the use of technology in sustaining life. In the social differentiation between legitimate and illegitimate intervention into the human body, social consensus declines if there is not a clear medical indication for the intervention. Where the patient is defined as 'terminally ill' and in need of palliative care, high technological interventions are viewed as 'unnatural' or 'artificial'. However, if the patient is defined as 'chronically ill' and her care is viewed as 'therapeutic', the distinction between health and disease is the line of social arbitration rather than the distinction between natural and unnatural. When medical technology is normalised through its assimilation of nature it is viewed as less threatening. Therefore, for example, if the feeding technology is presented as a source of nourishment, its application is justified as a natural right rather than as an invasion of bodily integrity. When the technology is withdrawn in the case of the former rationale there is a strong ethical argument that this is 'killing', whereas in the latter interpretation medical withdrawal is viewed as 'desistance'.

The public media coverage of the 'right to die' case shows how dominant cultural and social values underlie legal interpretations, and that legal decisions at the same time shape public debate. The courts defined the terms of reference of the individual case, which in turn became the key focus of the public construction of the debate. Within the time frame of the court rulings the media focus (in the main) was on mobilising a binary argumentation structure – representatives (medical, religious and theological experts) of two different world views: one which represented a traditional society was mobilised to legitimise the use of life-sustaining technology where the interests of the patient may conflict with medical opinion and practice, and the other as a representative of a modern society which asserts the right of the individual over the state and professional power.

The complexity of the issues concerning the terminally ill patient and the role of medical technology in terms of how it changes our normative conceptions of life and death, and the implications this has for subjective understandings of our bodies and for public policy in the regulation of medical practice, require a wider and more inclusive debate. For example, the rights of the family of the patient at the centre of the 'right to die' case and the significance of its experience had little visibility in the main time frame of the debate (see *The Irish Times*, 24 February 1996 and 6 March 1996). This is in part a reflection of the division between death as a private affair and death as a public issue which was foreshadowed in the discourse of the experts. Without a change in medical ethical guidelines and without a statutory response to the right to die case, the need for a public debate has since lost its momentum. Instead, the problem of the definition of death has been normalised as one which ultimately belongs to the sphere of scientific medicine, although individuals have the right to recourse to the law as an arbiter in the case of a conflict of interest. The broader implications of the role of medical technology in sustaining life and the medicalisation of the definition of death in the removal of organs from cadavers remained outside the terms of the debate. This, again, indicates the way in which legal frameworks can be strategically deployed to displace and fragment public interest and critique through 'discursive closure', i.e. the terms of the debate are already bound by the terms of reference of the key actors, which in this case are the legal and medical professions.

NRT and the Rights of the Infertile

For nearly two decades the NRT story has been sustained by public interest. This can be explained by the rapid rate of development of the technology which spawns social, ethical and legal dilemmas, solutions to which lag far behind technological possibilities. As the above discussion has emphasised, public interest is understood in the context of the growing politicisation of science in the light of rapid technological innovations in medicine. In Ireland, the construction of a public debate on NRT has changed significantly from the 1980s to the 1990s. In the early 1980s when AID was introduced as a service by the Well Woman Centre there was little sign of a public controversy about the potential use of the service by non-married couples, and single and lesbian women. When we examine the media coverage of the story, we find that there are only 'shadow' references to non-married, non-heterosexual recipients of AID. We can denote such shadow references by the way in which the dominant reference to the 'married couple' and the 'childless couple' negates the legitimacy of other potential clients. While single and lesbian women and, by the same token, non-married couples, are alluded to in the main press coverage given to the setting up of the service, they are not visible as legitimate subjects with distinct needs and claims. The 'married couple' is encoded in the medical definition of the need for an AID service. One newspaper article explains the need for the service in the following medical terms which foregrounds the potential recipient as the 'married couple': '. . . women whose husbands are infertile or whose sperm may carry a genetic disorder . . . where a woman with a Rhesus-negative blood group has already been sensitised by conceiving by a partner with Rhesus-positive blood. . .' (*The Irish Times*, 3 March 1982). Cultural assumptions are valorised as a way of avoiding open contestation over potentially competing claims about who should be able to avail of the service. The following quote reported from a representative of the WWC on the wider availability of its AID service illustrates this: 'I can't see these people being refused, but I don't know, the matter hasn't arisen yet. And I think AID is a fantastic answer for childless couples. You should see the change in them, once they have hope' (*The Irish Times*, 5 March 1982). The strategic avoidance of open contestation is evidenced by the way in which the need for AID is contextualised with reference to the falling number of babies available through adoption and the restrictions imposed by adoption laws for 'some couples'. The reference to adoption serves to reinforce cultural assumptions about the legitimacy of those who avail of AID, and at the same time it normalises the technology by appealing to the cultural investment in the genetic imperative of reproduction. The following newspaper quote illustrates how the physiology of pregnancy is evoked to naturalise the technology: '[the WWC] point out . . . that AID/AIH (Artificial Insemination by Husband) permits the parents to enjoy the process of pregnancy with the mother/child bonding that is absent in the case of adoption' (*Sunday Tribune*, 31 January 1981).

As mentioned earlier, the status of prospective children of AID is legally encoded in other countries. In Ireland there are no statutory provisions for children conceived through sperm donation. Instead, the status of the prospective child is assumed by the inevitability of the biological process and the arrangement of those facts within the context of marriage: '[t]he child when born, can be registered in the normal way and since the Well Woman Centre encourages couples to have sexual intercourse the night before insemination there is no way of knowing whether or not the father is in fact the husband' (*Sunday Tribune*, 31 January 1981) The anonymity of the donor, therefore, is protected not by legal principle, but by what is taken to be the normative context of the social organisation of sexual relations and 'father right'. The symbolic significance of the genetic imperative naturalises AID within existing cultural understandings of reproductive identity and its social organisation.

There was little significant media attention given to NRT practices in Ireland until the international media coverage of the postmenopausal birth phenomenon and other stories concerning the impregnation of a black woman with an embryo from a white woman, and reports sourced in the British media on clinical proposals on the use of eggs from aborted foetuses and eggs from cadavers in IVF procedures. Despite an earlier national newspaper article which reported on a self-imposed moratorium on IVF by the Irish medical profession, its introduction in 1989 received no significant coverage. In 1983 the assumed medical consensus on conceptive technology was framed in terms of abortion politics: '[t]he prevalent view in Irish medical circles is that human life begins as soon as fertilisation takes place in the laboratory and a human embryo has been formed . . .' (*Sunday Tribune*, 21 March 1983). The more intensive coverage of the issue in recent years does not explain what has changed to alter the moral consensus which effectively banned IVF technology. The international media exposure, at the juncture of 1993/1994, of the birth of twins to a 59 year-old British woman at the infamous Severino Antinori private fertility clinic in Rome was a key mobilising story in the construction of an Irish debate on NRT. While a debate ensued in relation to the need to regulate technologies which overstep cultural boundaries, the most salient concern to emerge was the protection against any diminution of the rights already conceded to childless couples.

In entering this public debate, the medical profession, conscious of how such stories had caught the public's imagination, had to subvert the moral discourse of the early 1980s. It did this by appealing to a new set of scientific facts and knowledge claims. The scientific rationale for more advanced fertility treatments is, in part, provided by scientific claims about the rising rate of infertility. Efficacy and cost benefit arguments which are used in oppositional discourses as an economic rationale for limiting resources in high technology such as IVF which has low success rates, are now recast in the context of a 'proven' need for such services to improve resource allocation for better and more efficient technologies. Furthermore, public fears which had been constructed around events elsewhere (the postmenopausal story and, more recently, the Mandy Allwood multiple pregnancy story and the destruction of thousands of frozen embryos in storage in British fertility clinics) are addressed in terms of the ethical guidelines of the Irish Medical Council which claim to preempt such controversies arising in the Irish context. However, reports such as the *Irish Independent* article (2 August 1985) with its caption 'Questions fall on fertile new ground: as this century comes to a close in vitro fertilisation could become the hottest topic here in Ireland', shows how the terms of the debate on NRT are shifting from the politics of moral insistence to a legalistic rationale and a discourse premised on the rights of the infertile.

The ethical restrictions which ban donor gametes and the freezing and storage of embryos, and the exclusion of non-married couples have themselves become the subject of public contestation. The mobilisation of NRT as a political issue has received its main impetus from the public launch in 1995 of a pressure group – The National Fertility Support and Information Group (NISIG). The key issues highlighted by the group are the social stigma of infertility, the failure of the medical profession to address the collective grievances of the infertile, the public information deficit on fertility treatments, the exercise of moral decisions by doctors which deny fertility patients an adequate knowledge base in the consultation process, and the implications of the present ethical limitations for the infertile. The use of personal narratives in the public media has become a discursive resource exploited by the NISIG to pursue fertility treatment as a rights issue. The construction of personal narratives as a public discourse strategy has increasingly entered popular representations of NRT. The subjective narrative is used to construct the 'need' for an expanding fertility service and the public visibility given to these biographical accounts is recast as a social commentary on the failure of the medical profession and the legislature to recognise the legitimacy of the needs of the infertile.

Medical regimes such as chemotherapy and their implications for fertility loss have led to a growing public awareness of the status of men's reproductive health. The personal narrative of a young Irish male who deposited sperm in a British sperm bank prior to chemotherapy treatment ('Banking on fatherhood', *The Irish Times*, 8 July 1996) is an account of the social processes involved in the changing status of sterility. This counter-narrative not only challenges social attitudes towards men and women's procreative identity, but also challenges what counts as legitimate medical knowledge and practice. Furthermore, it is an account of how meaning is constituted in human procreation and the exigent experiences of contemplating one's identity in a personal future which may well rule out the possibility of having genetic children of one's own. A growing constituency whose interest in a sperm bank facility is identified, i.e. men with Hodgkin's disease, leukaemia, testicular cancer, diabetes or multiple sclerosis. This relatively distinct constituency of potential 'users' whose needs are definable in terms of identifiable modern pathologies is aligned with a growing 'non-pathological' group of men whose fertility is negatively affected by environmental factors and the overall global trend in decreasing sperm counts. This broadens the definition of the problem and transforms the need idiom into a political discourse on rights, which in part is reflected by a growing network of interests publicly aligning themselves with the issue, including fertility clinics, and specialised public interest groups such as the Hodgkin's United Group.

The need for an expansive fertility service is communicated by the 'export script'. A *Sunday Times* article (18 August 1996) recounts the personal narrative of a fertility patient who has to travel outside the jurisdiction for IVF treatment involving donor sperm and reports on the case of a patient who died in 1995 following an illness after she received fertility treatment, again outside the jurisdiction. The export script which is a legacy of reproductive politics in Ireland is recast to highlight infertility as part of that political context: 'Generations of Irish women have left the country to buy contraceptives in Britain or Northern Ireland, or to undergo sterilisation and abortions, all prohibited at one time or another by law. A new generation is leaving for fertility treatment . . .' (*Sunday Times*, 18 August 1996).

The prospect of legal challenges to force a mandatory responsibility on the state is highlighted by the media announcement of prospective legal cases. The public announcement of an alliance between Bourne Hall – a private fertility clinic in Britain – and Clane Hospital to provide embryo freezing and storage which are ethically banned at present is explicitly framed as a mobilising strategy to force the pace of ethical and legislative change (RTÉ *Prime Time*, 24 October 1996). The issue of fertility treatment as a 'right' is being pursued through the alignment of legalistic and medical discourse frames. The fact that this is being brokered by an outside private clinic is, on the one hand, represented as an indictment on the Irish medical profession and, on the other hand, it serves to incorporate a market rationale on consumer choice and the need to protect clients in this unregulated market.

Conclusion

Both the debate on the 'right to die' case and the more extensive debate on NRT reminds us of the paradox of medical technology in the way in which it has (re)ordered the field of conception and death. While the encroachment of medical scientific knowledge into so many aspects of our lives implicates us further in the world of the profane, and medical technology makes it possible to reconstruct our bodies and the normative assumptions about biological contingency, this also leads to a crisis. This crisis manifests itself in the struggle over meaning. As the case studies above indicate, empirically there are different constructions (philosophical, social, ethical and legal) of the perceived and real problems engendered in medical technology. The concepts of 'artificial life' and 'artificial conception' express different visions, claims, and counter claims. Biomedical discourse is itself being reordered within such fields of conflict. As it engenders new objects and subjects of medicine, new potential fields of resistance emerge. However, as the case studies also show, the cultural assumptions which determine the application of medical technology – the ideology of progress, the rationality of diagnostic goals, the altruism of the doctor, etc. – are rarely questioned. Furthermore, the normative assumptions which are encoded in medical practice (for example, who are the recipients of the technology? who makes the decision?) continue to be governed by the self-regulatory sphere of the medical profession. The reluctance of the state to institutionalise a political mandate to, for example, the Supreme Court ruling in the 'right to die' case, or to legislate for infertility as a health status issue and to address the legal anomalies of NRT practices, leaves these questions within the governance of the self-regulatory sphere of medicine.

The normative issues raised by certain medical technologies are essentially public policy issues. The analytical or conceptual issues concern the very core values of human existence. For example, what is meaningful about having a genetic child of one's own? What is the meaning of death? How do shifts in our value structure affect subjective identities, collective understandings, and generative behaviour? These are some of the more salient issues which lie behind the social and ethical concerns raised by advances in medical technology.

Notes

I would like to recall here my gratitude to the late Dr Vincent Tucker for his insightful and encouraging comments on the first draft of this paper. Many thanks also to Dr Dolores Dooley for sharing her media bank on the Right to Die case.

1   The term 'discourse' will be used throughout this paper, and by discourse I mean the cultural construction of meaning: how meaning is established, communicated and interpreted.

2   Tony Bland suffered brain damage following the Hillsborough football disaster in Britain in 1989. His case was the first medico-legal dilemma in Britain concerning the request to terminate life support for a patient in a Persistent Vegetative State (PVS) discussed by the British House of Lords. The ruling in *Airedale NHS Trust v Bland* (see Tomkin and Hanafin, 1995: 157–8) shows how medical practice is structured by the nature of the relationship between culture and technology, and how this relationship is increasingly mediated by a discourse on rights, i.e. the rights of patients.

3   The problem of definition over an illness category, which for example arose in the 'right to die' case concerning the question of whether the patient was in a persistent vegetative state or a 'near' persistent vegetative state, is not simply a question of scientific calculation; social values also play a role in 'scientific' judgements.

4   Economic rationalisation is increasingly accepted as a legitimate basis for state intervention in the delivery of health care. The rationing of limited health resources, however, is not an uncontested issue ethically, socially or politically. When it comes to the health status of the terminally ill, 'cost consciousness' proves particularly contentious for public representatives. Advances in medical knowledge and technology, decreasing public resources and increasing demand for an ever-widening range of treatments creates the conditions of conflict over health status. The simplistic rationale of demand and supply equally proves contentious when, for example, we consider the changing face of health and illness from acute to chronic illness and the growth in the numbers affected by terminal illness.

References

Corea, G. (1988) *The Mother Machine: Reproductive Technologies from Artificial Insemination to Artificial Wombs*. London: Women's Press.

Habermas, J. (1991) *The Theory of Communicative Action. Vol. 1: Reason and the Rationalization of Society*, Cambridge: Polity.

Harrison, R. (1992) An Irish out-patient based in-vitro fertilisation service, *Irish Medical Journal*, 85(2): 63–5.

Kaplan, L. J. and R. Tong (1994) *Controlling Our Reproductive Destiny: A Technological and Philosophical Perspective*. Cambridge: MIT Press.

Lupton, D. (1994) *Medicine as Culture: Illness, Disease and the Body in Western Societies*, London: Sage.

Martin, E. (1993) *The Woman in the Body*. Milton Keynes: Open University Press.

Medical Council (1994) *Constitution and Functions: A Guide to Ethical Conduct and Behaviour, and to Fitness to Practise* (4th edition) Dublin: Medical Council.

Outhwaite, W. (ed.) (1996) *The Habermas Reader*. Cambridge: Polity.

Price, F (1993) Beyond expectation: clinical practices and clinical concerns, in: J. Edwards and S. Franklin (eds) *Technologies of Procreation: Kinship in the Age of Assisted Conception*. Manchester: Manchester University Press.

Stanworth, M. (ed.) (1987) *Reproductive Technologies: Gender, Motherhood and Medicine*. Cambridge: Polity.

Tomkin, D. and P. Hanafin (1995) *Irish Medical Law*. Dublin: Round Hall Press.

Turner, B. S. (1992a) *Medical Power and Social Knowledge*. London: Sage.

Turner, B. S. (1992b) *Regulating Bodies: Essays in Medical Sociology*. London: Routledge.

Section 2

INEQUALITIES IN HEALTH CARE

5

Social Class Differences in Some Lifestyle and Health Characteristics in Ireland

Lessons from a Coronary Heart Disease Community Health Promotion Programme

Claire Collins and Emer Shelley

The relationship between health and social class has been documented since the nineteenth century. The Black Report (DHSS, 1980), however, gave impetus to the discussion and has prompted many investigations and reviews. Research in many countries has shown that social class is an accurate predictor of mortality and there is growing evidence that social habits are related to health and morbidity patterns. According to Graham and Reeder (1979), 'Social class or socio-economic status can be related to all illness and health in general'. Social class not only points to a differential life span but also a difference in the experience of illness throughout life. Power (1994) in his review of health and social inequality in Europe stated that 'it is almost universally the case that people in lower social classes have more morbidity and disability and have shorter lives'.

In additon to the existence of health inequalities, much work has been published outlining possible explanations for the relationship. The main explanations discussed have been selective drift, materialist/social, cultural/ behavioural, artefact, physical environment, access to services and biological inheritance (DHSS, 1980; Smith *et al*, 1990; Power, 1994). It has been shown that a combination of these factors prevails and that intervention needs to consider the interaction between factors in addition to addressing the independent effects.

Commitment to the reduction of inequalities has been formalised in European agreements and various strategies have been employed in other countries to this end. The World Health Organisation European strategy for 'Health for All' includes the target that 'by the year 2000, the actual differences in health status between countries and between groups within countries should be reduced by at least 25%, by improving the level of disadvantaged nations and groups.' (WHO, 1986).

The Department of Health in Ireland has recognised the determining effect of socio-economic factors on health (1994; 1995). However, the 'Health Promotion Strategy' document (1995) points to the scarcity of information on variations in health status according to socio-economic group. Research has consistently demonstrated the relationship between socio-economic position and various aspects of health, such as health status, health behaviour and perceptions of health. Data specific to the Irish situation, although not extensive, is covincing and consistent with international findings.

Nolan (1990) found significant differences in standardised mortality rates between the professional/managerial groups and the semi-skilled/unskilled groups in Ireland. The rates were comparable with those in England and Wales although a steeper gradient was observed between the Irish groups. Johnson and Lyons's work (1993) support Nolan's findings and conclude that there is a relationship between mortality and socio-eonomic indicators in Dublin with higher mortality in disadvantaged areas. Inequalities related to social class, gender and region have also been demonstrated with respect to diseases, such as respiratory diseases, heart attacks, cancer and pneumonia (Cook, 1990; Dean, 1982).

The largest category of deaths in Ireland is that caused by cardiovascular disease, mainly heart disease and stroke. Within cardiovascular diseases, the largest proportion of deaths are due to coronary heart disease (CHD). Mortality from CHD has been declining slowly in Irish men aged 30–69 years since 1974 and in Irish women in this age range since the 1950s. The rates of decline compare unfavourably with those in other countries and mortality from CHD in Ireland remains high by Western European standards. The findings of the Kilkenny Health Project (KHP) highlight the existence of social class differences in Ireland in lifestyle and health characteristics relevant to CHD and the persistence of these differences over time despite overall improvements in the health of the population. The use of this data to further the discussion on health and social class in Ireland is considered appropriate given that cardiovascular disease accounts for 30% of premature deaths in Ireland (Department of Health, 1994) and because many of the factors related to CHD morbidity and mortality are also relevant to other illness and control of CHD risk factors could lead to a reduction in other diseases.

The KHP was established in 1985 due to a concern with the lack of parallel between falling rates of CHD mortality in Ireland and such countries as America, Canada, Finland and Australia. The overall aim of the KHP was to implement and evaluate a community-based programme to reduce coronary heart disease. The Project involved a two stage survey process with baseline and follow-up data collected in 1985/86 and 1990/91 respectively in an intervention and reference county. An independent, geographically clustered, stratified random sample of the population in each county in each of the two time periods was chosen by the RANSAM programme (Whelan, 1979). Details on the methods employed have been reported elsewhere (Shelley *et al.*, 1995). The data presented are from a sub-study of the KHP which involved a five-year follow-up of the respondents who participated in the survey in the intervention county (Co. Kilkenny) in 1985.

There were 792 respondents interviewed in 1985. These respondents were followed up in 1990 and requested to take part in a follow-up survey. In 1990, 709 of these respondents were interviewed. The response rate was 78.3% in 1985 of whom 89% were re-interviewed in 1990. The data analysis is based on the 686 respondents who were interviewed in both surveys and for whom social class data were recorded.

The social class breakdown of the respondents compared to the social class distribution for Co. Kilkenny and Ireland is shown in Table 1. The percentage of respondents in social classes 1 and 2 is higher than the percentages in these classes in Co. Kilkenny and Ireland (Census Report, 1986). The percentage of the survey population in classes 4 to 6 is lower than the same percentage for the Kilkenny and National populations.

Table 1 *Social class of respondents*

Social Class	Survey population N	Survey population %	Kilkenny population %	National population %
1	89	13.0	9.7	11.0
2	185	27.0	18.5	15.7
3	127	18.5	18.3	19.5
4	152	22.2	26.4	25.3
5	71	10.3	14.6	17.1
6	62	9.0	12.4	11.4
Total	686	100.0	100.0	100.0

Table 2 presents the data for mean total serum cholesterol, mean systolic and diastolic blood pressure and prevalence of obesity for the social classes in 1985 and 1990.

The results did not show an association between social class and mean serum total cholesterol in either the first (1985) or second (1990) survey. The highest value in 1985 was for social class 6 (6.18 mmol/l) and in 1990 was for social class 1 (6.03 mmol/l); however, the level was similar at approximately 6.0 mmol/l for all groups. One would expect cholesterol to increase with age. The figures revealed that, although the respondents were five-years older,

Table 2 *Comparison of health characteristics between the social classes*

	Social Class 1	Social Class 2	Social Class 3	Social Class 4	Social Class 5	Social Class 6
Mean total serum cholesterol (mmol/l)						
1985	6.12	5.99	6.09	5.95	6.02	6.18
1990	6.03	5.97	5.97	5.97	5.77	5.90
Mean systolic BP (mmHg)						
1985	139.3	139.7	142.9	139.8	145.6	146.8
1990	137.8	137.8	139.8	139.7	141.6	146.2
Mean diastolic BP (mmHg)						
1985	77.2	76.6	77.6	76.9	79.4	81.3
1990	77.8	76.9	77.2	78.0	78.5	81.0
Obesity (%)						
1985	15.7	7.0	13.4	12.5	16.9	27.4
1990	23.6	8.1	14.2	17.8	19.7	25.8

mean cholesterol levels were lower in 1990. The most substantial changes were in classes 5 (0.25 mmol/l) and 6 (0.28 mmol/l).

The mean SBP figures for the social classes showed an overall gradient. The highest SBP level was in social class 6, 146.8 mmHg in 1985 and 146.2 mmHg in 1990, and the lowest was in social class 1, 139.3 mmHg in 1985 and 137.8 mmHg in 1990. The results for mean DBP exhibited the same trend, social class 6 had the highest level, 81.3 and 81.0 mmHg in 1985 and 1990 respectively and social class 1 had the lowest level, 77.2 mmHg in 1985 and 77.8 mmHg in 1990. The level of SBP decreased for all classes, despite the respondents being five years older, with the greatest changes being in classes 3 and 5. Although the levels remained higher in the manual social classes, the gap between the classes narrowed. The changes in DBP showed no discernible pattern with the levels for classes 1, 3, 5 and 6 having decreased and the levels for classes 2 and 4 having increased, although the increase is not of the same magnitude that might usually be expected given the age increase of respondents.

The results in 1985 and 1990 showed a similar pattern with exceptionally high proportions of social classes 1 and 6 being obese, and a comparatively low prevalence of obesity in class 2. The percentage of respondents classified as obese increased for all classes between 1985 and 1990, except social class 6 where a decrease of 1.6% was noted. The increase was greatest in classes 1 (7.9%) and 4 (5.3%).

Table 3 compares the social classes in terms of their prevalence of smoking and alcohol consumption, weekly exercise and level of knowledge about CHD factors.

Table 3 *Comparison of lifestyle characteristics between the social classes*

	Social Class 1	Social Class 2	Social Class 3	Social Class 4	Social Class 5	Social Class 6
Current Smokers						
1985	25.8	25.5	20.5	34.9	40.8	53.2
1990	22.4	22.2	22.8	28.3	38.0	40.3
Alcohol Drinkers						
1985	79.8	68.7	71.7	69.7	69.0	71.0
1990	77.5	70.3	70.1	69.7	64.8	70.9
Mean units of alcohol per week						
1985	11.7	12.2	10.4	9.8	20.5	18.0
1990	10.3	11.9	10.7	9.6	17.9	17.8
Light exercise twice or more per week						
1985	24.7	30.4	22.8	28.3	22.5	27.4
1990	55.1	62.7	56.7	55.9	67.6	56.5
Good level of knowledge about CHD factors						
1985	67.4	63.8	53.5	52.6	39.4	30.7
1990	84.3	70.2	69.3	56.6	50.7	53.2

The 1985 data show significant differences between the percentage of smokers in each social class. The percentage of smokers decreased slightly from class 1 (25.8%) to class 3 (20.5%) and then increased sharply in class 4 (34.9%) and further to class 6 (53.2%). Approximately twice as many people in the manual social classes smoked as people in the non-manual groups. The 1990 data also showed a significant relationship between smoking status and social class membership. Comparing the percentage of smokers in each class in 1985 and 1990 showed that the percentage decreased in all but one social class grouping – the proportion of smokers in social class 3 increased by 2%. The change was most substantial in classes 4 and 6, with a decrease of 6.6% in class 4 and 12.9% in class 6.

Analysis of the alcohol consumption of the social classes did not show a significant relationship between social class membership and alcohol consumption status. The percentage of current alcohol drinkers in each social class varied very little except for the slightly larger percentage found in social class 1, 79.8% in 1985 and 77.5% in 1990. Current drinkers in social classes 5 and 6 had the highest mean intake of alcohol per week, while those in classes 3 and 4 had the lowest mean intake. The mean units of alcohol consumed per week by current drinkers were substantially higher in classes 5 and 6 than in any other group and this difference persisted across the time period of the surveys. The changes in the percentage of current alcohol drinkers in each social class were small. The greatest reduction was in social class 5 (4.2%). A reduction of approximately 10% was noted in the mean units of alcohol consumed per week with a decrease of 1.4 units for social class 1 and 2.6 units for social class 6.

There was no significant difference between the classes with regard to light exercise activities. Only 26.7% of the respondents in 1985 reported exercising two or more times per week, the lowest percentage was for class 5 (22.5%), the highest was for class 2 (30.4%). In 1990, the percentage of respondents exercising two or more times per week was highest in social class 5 (67.6%) and lowest in social class 1 (55%). The percentage for social class 2 was also high with 63.7% of social class 2 repondents exercising two or more times per week. There were substantial increases in activity levels between the surveys. The percentage exercising doubled in each social class group. The increase for classes 1 to 3 was 30% while the figures for classes 4 and 6 were marginally lower at 27.6% and 29% respectively. Social class 5 had the largest increase in the proportion of its members taking exercise (45%).

There were significant differences between the social classes in the level of knowledge about health and CHD risk factors. The results show that the lower classes compared badly with the other classes in terms of knowledge. In 1985, 67.4% of social class 1 respondents possessed a good level of knowledge about health issues. The percentage was slightly lower for social class 2 respondents (63.8%). The percentage for social classes 3 and 4 was lower at 53.5% and 52.6% respectively. Social classes 5 and 6 were much less well informed with 39.4% of class 5 and 30.6% of class 6 members having a good level of knowledge about factors which affect their health. Although the percentages were higher in 1990, the data revealed similar trends. The percentage for social class 1 was 84.3% and this decreased to 53.2% in class 6. The percentage of class members with a good level of knowledge about the factors which affect coronary heart disease increased for all social classes between 1985 and 1990. The increase was greatest for classes 6 (22.6%), 1 (16.8%) and 3 (15.7%). The increases in classes 2 (6.4%) and 4 (3.9%) were small in comparison.

The data show an association with social class for smoking prevalence, alcohol consumption, prevalence of obesity, mean SBP, mean DBP and knowledge levels but not for mean total cholesterol or light leisure activity. The effect of social class remained when age and sex were controlled. Studies in other countries which have also investigated variation in CHD mortality and risk factor levels have concluded that one's social position has a strong predictive value. The Happy Heart National Survey carried out in 1992 showed similar differences in current smoking, current alcohol consumption and obesity between the manual and non-manual classes at the National level (Irish Heart Foundation, 1994).

The KHP data is of particular value in that it provides the opportunity to observe trends over time. There is evidence that absolute risk factor levels have declined and that the relative position of the manual social classes (classes 4–6) has improved slightly, although these classes remained in a less well-off position with regard to lifestyle and health characteristics. The prevalence levels and the changes over time observed in the KHP data are similar to those reported by other studies, both in Ireland and elsewhere.

Over the five years of the Project, changes were observed in health status as measured by CHD risk factors. These changes varied in magnitude by social class, age, and sex. The KHP showed decreased levels of CHD risk factors between 1985 and 1990. The changes which were recorded are consistent with the findings internationally. Luepker *et al.* (1993), reporting on risk factor trends from the Minnesota Heart Survey, conclude that the lower social groups continue to have the highest level of risk characteristics and CHD rates. McLoone and Boddy (1994) found an increasing distinction between the classes between 1981 and 1991 in Scotland with respect to mortality and Phillimore *et al.* (1994) showed that mortality differentials in Northern England widened between 1981 and 1991. The persistence of such disparities highlights the social determination of disease (Susser *et al.*, 1983).

The KHP findings show an overall gradient between the manual (classes 4–6) and non-manual (classes 1–3) groups. However, the variation between classes within this distinction suggests that a multiplicity of factors are relevant to the explanation of health inequalities.

The independent effect of the KHP community programme is difficult to distinguish. Firstly, the possible existence of lag-time means that changes prompted by the Project may not have taken effect in such a short period. Secondly, major shifts were occurring nationally during the time of the Project and finally, it was difficult to avoid cross-border 'contamination', from the use of national television for example. It is for this last reason that the data for the reference county are not presented. In addition, it is of interest to note that there were some disparities observed between the findings of the 'cohort' (1985 respondents re-interviewed in 1990) and the independent survey of 1990 in the intervention county. This was exhibited in the fact that the overall changes led to an increased disparity between the classes in the independent survey and a slightly decreased disparity between the classes in the cohort survey. This may in some part be due to the fact that the respondent's GP was notified if the respondent had high blood pressure, cholesterol etc.

The lessons learnt by the KHP and the materials developed by them would benefit any national programme to affect health and lifestyle changes within Ireland.

The findings of the KHP suggest that education alone is insufficient to improve the relative position of the manual social classes. Conroy *et al.* (1986)

provided support for this and concluded that the lower social class failed to maintain change and exhibited low levels of compliance although they appeared equally well informed. Many sociologists have identified the cultural context in which illness occurs as important and Conroy (1994), in his qualitative investigation in a small Irish community, suggests that it is not the lack of knowledge but a lack of awareness of the importance of CHD as a health problem and disbelief that personal actions could affect one's life span. Of paramount importance to the success of educational programmes is the ability to communicate messages to the population, particularly the socially and economically disadvantaged. Transmission methods to reach the desired population and language which can be understood by these individuals is of particular importance (Collins *et al.*, 1993).

One must recognise that people live differently and that how one lives, what one thinks, and how one behaves are crucial in determining one's attitude to health and indeed one's susceptibility to illness. Green and Johnson propound that 'health behavior and responses to health education are correlated with specific beliefs concerning personal susceptibility and severity of consequences, the efficacy of recommended practices and with beliefs concerning whether health is an outcome under a person's control' (1983). Individuals must therefore be convinced of their susceptibility to illness and of their ability to influence it.

The social structure of a society exerts an influence on the health of the members of that society. Cockerham believed that 'on nearly every measure membership in lower social classes carries health penalties . . . To be poor is by definition to have less of the things (including health care) produced by society' (1978). The underlying cause of this deprivation is not solely material. The implications of membership of a particular class are not only economic but feed into all aspects of one's existence. One's attitudes, beliefs and lifestyle are all affected by the social class to which one belongs.

> I think it's a pretty serious and important factor to the extent that we have a good deal of evidence to show that, right from the beginning of life, one's life chances, the chance of surviving birth, of suffering from certain illnesses, the chances of living in certain types of accommodation, of receiving certain types of education and indeed the likelihood of earning a given income, are very much related to divisions in our society which we call social class. In fact, there seems to be very little of life in our society which isn't in some way characterised by differences between social classes. (Reid, 1989).

One must define health and establish what it means to people and how it affects their lives. Green and Johnson (1983) summarise that 'the social influence of occupational, educational, and economic identity shape attitudes toward health, illness, and behaviour concerning both health and illness'.

The evidence on the success of different interventions suggest that a combination of high risk and population approaches is appropriate.

The results from the Swedish Community Intervention Programme showed that the ability to obtain knowledge and utilise information was socially stratified and thus Brannstrom *et al.* (1993) recommend that a selected preventive strategy might be more effective than community-oriented approaches which appear to contribute to the widening of inequalities. Syme and Guralnik (1987) stress that there is logic in focusing not on particular risk factors but on an integrated approach dealing with high risk groups due to the synergistic effect of risk factors. They suggest that the greatest potential for future policy may lie in a more balanced approach which gives attention to community and ecological approaches. Shelley (1994) emphasised that 'priority should be given to health promotion initiatives which make the environment more conducive to health-enhancing lifestyles'. Delamothe (1991) recognised the limitations on initiatives to reduce individual risk factors imposed by the absence of a wider strategy to reduce deprivation and improve the environment.

Whitehead *et al.* (1993) outlined the pioneering attempts made in Australia to tackle social inequalities in health. The success in Australia can be attributed to the fact that inequality issues were taken seriously, targets and goals were set and advice and participation were encouraged from many sectors. The concentration on specific social groups and on formulating targets for the wider social and environmental determinants of health and the inclusion of the equity audit of the health care sector are the major strengths of the Australian initiatives.

The World Health Organisation (1988) recommends that 'All nations . . . should pursue further targets of improvement of the health of all their people so as to ensure that every citizen has the opportunity to live a socially and economically productive life'. Among the key principles of 'Health for All' are the ideas of equity, effectiveness, and intersectoral collaboration. It is necessary that we address ourselves to these issues and create an environment which is conducive to healthy living for the entire population. Finally, if 'Health for All' is to be achieved it is necessary to place health promotion and health policy in a wider social context and to encourage cooperation between professionals.

Appendix to chapter 5

Social class was defined on the basis of occupation for this analysis and was measured using the Irish Census based socio-economic group classification system. This scale groups the census occupational units into six discrete ordinal class categories on the basis of their market and work situations (Figure 1). The classification 'has a validity in an Irish context beyond that of alternative scales . . .' (O'Hare *et al.*, 1991). While reservations exist about the use of this single factor, it proves to be an appropriate tool. Monk (1970) argued that 'Occupation remained the backbone of social grading because no better methods have been found, and because it has still remained a powerful and useful stratification factor'.

Figure 1
Irish census-based social class classifications

Social class 1:   Higher professional, higher managerial, proprietors and farmers farming 200+ acres.

Social class 2:   Lower professional, lower managerial, proprietors and farmers farming 100–199 acres.

Social class 3:   Other non-manual and farmers farming 50–99 acres.

Social class 4:   Skilled manual and farmers farming 30–49 acres.

Social class 5:   Semi-skilled manual and farmers farming < 30 acres.

Social class 6:   Unskilled manual.

The World Health Organization MONICA (**Moni**toring Trends and Determinants in **C**ardiovascular Disease) project smoking categorisations are used to summarise the data obtained on smoking practices in the survey population. Current smokers smoke at least one cigarette daily, 1g or more of pipe tobacco daily or 1 cigar or more per week. Those who quit smoking within the month prior to the survey were also categorised as current smokers.

Current alcohol drinkers were respondents who consumed any quantity of beer, wine or spirits in the year preceding the survey interview.

Body mass index (BMI) is an expression of the size of an individual taking height into account (BMI = weight/height^2, Kg/m^2). The respondent was considered in the acceptable weight category where BMI was < 25.0, overweight where BMI was 25.0–< 30.0 and obese where BMI was 30.0+.

Total serum cholesterol was estimated using the CHOD-PAP enzymatic colorimetric method of Boehringer Mannheim. Total serum cholesterol is reported as mmol/L.

A Hawksley Random Zero Sphygmomanometer with random zero 0–20 mmHg was used to measure blood pressure. The systolic blood pressure (SBP) and diastolic blood pressure (DBP) were recorded to the nearest 2 millimaters of mercury (mmHg). The measurement was taken twice and the mean of the two measurements reported.

Physical activity outside of work is reported. Light activity causes one to become a little short of breath and to perspire; it includes walking to and from work, gardening and dancing. Vigorous activity includes activity with shortness of breath, rapid heart rate and sweating for at least twenty minutes weekly.

Knowledge about health was derived by combining the answers received to thirteen questions. A scale was created based on the number of correct answers and respondents were classified as having 'little or no knowledge', 'a moderate level of knowledge' or ' a good level of knowledge'.

Acknowledgements

Sincere thanks are extended to all the respondents who took part in the Kilkenny Health Project and to the Project staff without whom the data would never have been collected. The Kilkenny Health Project was supported by the Department of Health, the Irish Heart Foundation and the South Eastern Health Board. Evaluation was overseen by a Scientific Committee chaired by Professor Ian Graham. Statistical support was provided by Dr Leslie Daly.

References

Blane D., G.D. Smith and M. Bartly (1990) Social class differences in years of potential life lost: size, trends, and principal causes, *British Medical Journal*, 301, 429–32.

Brannstrom I., L. Weinehall, L.A. Persson, P.O. Wester and S. Wall (1993) Changing social patterns of risk factors for cardiovascular disease in a Swedish community intervention programme, *International Journal of Epidemiology*, 22: 1026–37.

Central Statistics Office. 1986. *Census 1986*. Dublin: Stationery Office.

Cockerham W.C. (1978) *Medical Sociology*. New Jersey: Prentice-Hall.

Collins C., L. Daly and E. Shelley (1993) Penetration of the Kilkenny Health Project education programme, *HYGIE*, XII: 11–13.

Conroy R.M. (1994) Culture, health beliefs and attitudes in a rural Irish community, *Anthropology Ireland*, 4 (1): 22–32.

Conroy R.M. *et al.* (1986) The relation of social class to risk factors, rehabilitation, compliance and mortality in survivors of acute coronary heart disease, *Scandinavian Journal of Social Medicine*, 14: 51–6.

Cook G. (1990) Health and social inequities in Ireland, *Social Science and Medicine*, 31 (3): 285–90.

Dean G. (1982) Respiratory disease and heart attacks among rural workers in Ireland and other countries of the European Economic Community, *Irish Medical Journal*, 75 (9): 338–42.

Delamothe T. (1991) Social inequalities in health, *British Medical Journal*, 303: 1046–50.

Department of Health (1994) *Shaping a Healthier Future*. Dublin: Department of Health

Department of Health. (1995) *A Health Promotion Strategy*. Dublin: Department of Health.

Department of Health (1995) *A Guide to Daily Healthy Food Choices*. Dublin: Health Promotion Unit, leaflet.

DHSS (Department of Health and Social Security) (1980) *Inequalities in Health: Report of a Research Working Group*. London: DHSS.

Graham S. and L.G. Reeder (1979) Social Epidemiology of Chronic Dieases. in: Freeman, Levine, Reeder, *Handbook of Medical Sociology*, 3rd edition. New Jersey: Prentice-Hall: 71–97.

Green L .W. and K.W. Johnson (1983) Health education and health promotion in D. Mechanic (ed.), *Handbook of Health, Health Care, and the Health Professions*. New York: The Free Press.

Haralambos M. and M. Holborn (1991) *Sociology, Themes and Perspectives*, 3rd edition. London: Collins.

Irish Heart Foundation (1994) *Happy Heart National Survey: A Report on Health Behaviour in Ireland*. Dublin: Irish Heart Foundation.

Johnson Z. And R. Lyons (1993) Socioeconomic factors and mortality in small areas, *Irish Medical Journal*, 86 (2): 60–2.

Luepker R.V., W.D. Rosamond, R. Murphy *et al.* (1983) Socioeconomic status and coronary heart disease risk factor trends. The Minnesota heart survey, *Circulation*, 88: 2172–9.

McLoone P. and F.A. Boddy (1994) Deprivation and mortality in Scotland, 1981 and 1991, *British Medical Journal*, 309: 1465–70.

Monk D. (1970) *Social Grading on the National Readership Survey*. London: Joint Industry Committee for National Readership Surveys.

Nolan B. (1990) Socio-economic mortality differentials in Ireland, *Economic and Social Review*, 21: 193–208.

O'Hare A., C.T. Whelan and P. Commins (1991) Development of an Irish census-based social class scale, *Economic and Social Review*, 22: 135–56.

Phillimore P, A. Beattie and P. Townsend (1994) Widening inequality of health in Northern England, 1981–91, *British Medical Journal*, 308: 1125–8.

Power C. (1994) Health and social inequality in Europe, *British Medical Journal*, 308: 1153–6.

Reid I. (1989) *Social Class Differences in Britain: Life Chances and Lifestyles*, 3rd edition. London: Fontana.

Shelley E. (1994) Can community programmes promote heart healthy lifestyles? *The Irish Journal of Psychology*, 15 (1): 164–78.

Shelley E., L. Daly and C. Collins *et al.* (1995) Cardiovascular risk factor changes in the Kilkenny Health Project. A community health promotion programme, *European Heart Journal*, 16: 752–60.

Smith G.D., M. Bartley and D. Blane (1990) The Black Report on socioeconomic inequalities in health 10 years on, *British Medical Journal*, 301: 373–7.

Susser M., K. Hopper and J. Richman (1983) Society, culture and health, in: D. Mechanic (ed.) *Handbook of Health, Health Care, and the Health Professions*. New York: The Free Press.

Syme S.L. and J.M. Guralnik (1987) Epidemiology and health policy: coronary heart disease, in S. Levine and A. Lilienfeld (eds), *Epidemiology and Health Policy*. New York and London: Tavistock.

Whelan B.J. (1979) RANSAM: a random sample design for Ireland, *Economic and Social Review*, 10: 169–74.

Whitehead M. and G. Dahlgren (1991) What can be done about inequalities in health? *The Lancet*, 338: 1059–63.

Whitehead M., K. Judge, D.J. Hunter, R. Maxwell and M.A. Scheuer (1993) Tackling inequalities in health: the Australian experience. *British Medical Journal*, 306: 783–7.

WHO (World Health Organisation) (1986) *Targets for Health for All. Targets in Support of the European Regional Strategy for Health for All*. Copenhagen: WHO.

WHO (World Health Organisation). (1988) *Priority Research for Health for All*. Copenhagen: WHO Regional Office for Europe.

WHO (World Health Organisation). (1989) MONICA Project. WHO MONICA Project: Objectives and design, *International Journal of Epidemiology*, 3 (Supplement): S29–S39.

6

Unemployment and Health

Brian Nolan and Christopher T. Whelan

Introduction

Our objective in this chapter is to set out briefly what is known about the relationship between unemployment and ill-health. We use evidence for Ireland where possible, but also draw on research carried out in Britain, the USA and elsewhere. The relationship between unemployment and ill-health is a complex and much-studied one. Cross-section studies have shown that in general unemployed people have poorer health than those who are in jobs (e.g. Warr, 1987), but this sort of evidence has to be interpreted with care. This does not necessarily mean that unemployment itself *causes* this ill-health. Obviously, it could work the other way around: illness could itself be contributing to the difficulties someone is having in the labour market. Serious or frequent illness could make it difficult for an individual to get a good education or to get and keep a 'good' job. In addition to looking at the association between unemployment and ill-health, then, we are also interested in the causal processes at work, and it may not be easy to tease out the direction of the effects.

An alternative avenue of research has been to look at how mortality and unemployment have varied over time, as in the work by Brenner (1979, 1983) which generated a substantial debate in the literature. He concluded that mortality rates in England and the USA were significantly related to earlier unemployment rates, but this provoked considerable controversy about methodological issues and interpretation (see for example the papers in Smith, 1987). Subsequent work has made clear that it is important not to focus too narrowly on the relationship between being unemployed and being ill, without looking at the background structural factors which mean that both unemployment and ill-health are more likely to be experienced by certain types of people, from particular socio-economic backgrounds or environments. We will therefore also say something about the broad relationship between health and social class, to provide this context.

Thirdly, it is helpful to distinguish between physical and psychological ill-health: although they may interact with each other, it appears that there may be important differences between the two in the nature of the relationship with unemployment. We will discuss first physical health before turning to unemployment and psychological health.

Physical Ill-Health

The Black Report, published in 1980, put health inequalities 'on the map' in Britain, and has been influential in winning wider attention for the issue in other countries. It documented the fact that there were large differentials in both mortality and morbidity favouring the higher social classes, and that these had persisted over time despite improvements in health and social services. The most striking evidence related to mortality: around 1971 the death rate for men aged between 15 and 64 was almost twice as high for those in the bottom (unskilled manual) class as in the top (professional and managerial) one. Subsequent British data suggest that these differentials if anything widened rather than narrowed up to 1981. The basis for these findings is the comparison of information from death certificates, which include occupation, with Census data on the total numbers in each occupational group or social class.

Some recent research for the Republic of Ireland (Nolan, 1990) using the same type of approach and methods has shown similar substantial differentials across socio-economic groups. (SEGs). Since the death rate for each SEG for the entire 15–64 age group will be influenced by its age composition, it is useful to look at death rates within narrower age groups. Table 1 shows, for example, that in the 55–64 age range the death rate for the higher professional group is 13 per 1,000 compared with 22 for the semi-skilled manual and 32 for the unskilled manual groups. Similarly, in the 45–54 range the rate per 1,000 for unskilled manual workers is 11 compared with that of 4 for higher professionals.

Alternatively, summary measures for the entire 15–64 age range that *standardise* for the differing age composition of the SEGs can be calculated. Standardised mortality ratios (SMRs) designed to do this are commonly used in the literature in this context. These involve calculating what the expected number of deaths for a particular SEG would be if the population in that SEG in each age range – 25–34, 35–44 etc. – experienced the average death rate over all SEGs for that age range. The actual total of deaths for the SEG is then expressed as a percentage of the expected deaths. An SMR over 100 thus means that the SEG had more deaths than would be expected on the

Table 1 *Mortality Rates for Men Aged 15–64 by Socio-economic Group, Ireland 1981*

Socio-economic Group	15–24	25–34	35–44	45–54	55–64	Standardised Mortality Rate
			death rate per 1,000			
Farmers	0.9	0.8	1.4	5.6	14.8	79
Farm labourers	1.6	1.3	3.1	4.6	15.2	86
Higher professional	0.2	0.3	0.8	3.5	12.8	55
Lower professional	1.5	0.5	1.4	5.5	16.0	79
Employers and managers	0.9	0.5	1.2	4.5	11.6	62
Salaried employees	1.0	0.6	1.5	3.6	15.2	71
Non-manual white collar	1.0	1.1	2.4	7.8	20.2	105
Non-manual other	1.8	1.2	2.0	6.2	20.1	104
Skilled manual	0.9	0.7	1.9	6.2	18.7	91
Semi-skilled manual	1.7	1.1	3.0	7.2	22.1	117
Unskilled manual	1.9	1.5	3.4	10.7	31.6	163
Unknown	3.0	6.8	6.8	13.4	25.9	174

basis of its age profile. Table 1 shows that, for men aged 15–64, the standardised mortality rate in 1981 was three times as great for the unskilled manual group as for the higher professional group – 163 as against 55. The group for whom occupation is 'unknown' had an even higher mortality rate than the unskilled manual group. Information on occupation is particularly likely to be missing for those who were unemployed for a considerable period, while unskilled manual workers experience much more unemployment than the other identified groups. Lower socio-economic status is therefore associated with both more unemployment experience and considerably higher mortality rates than for other groups. Skilled manual groups have an SMR close to 100 and for intermediate groups of non-manual workers they are just about 100.

Again, the causation could run from health to unemployment and socio-economic status rather than vice versa, with ill-health leading individuals with a high risk of dying to move down or remain towards the bottom of the socio-economic hierarchy. This is not something one could prove or disprove by looking at data of this type. However, recent research using a British longitudinal database which has information for *the same* individuals for 1971 and 1981 has shown that health-related social mobility of this kind does not account for the observed mortality differentials between the classes (Goldblatt, 1989; Fox, Goldblatt and Jones, 1986).

The same British data also allowed researchers to focus specifically on the mortality between 1971 and 1981 of men who were unemployed in 1971. This showed that mortality among this group was even higher than would be expected on the basis of their social class composition – unemployment at the starting-date was itself associated with 'excess' mortality even given broader social class effects (Moser, Fox and Jones 1986). Again, this did not seem to be explained by selection effects.

We now turn from mortality to morbidity. The Black report had little data on morbidity, but since then a good deal of information on differentials across social classes in Britain has become available from general household surveys and special health and lifestyles surveys. For example, the annual General Household Survey shows about 25% of professional men aged 16–64 reporting a long-standing illness, compared with about 40% of unskilled manual men.

Similar information on self-reported long-standing illness was obtained for the Republic in the household survey carried out by the Economic and Social Research Institute (ESRI) in 1987. As Table 2 shows, the percentage of adults reporting such illness was at least twice as high for the unskilled manual as for the professional and managerial classes (Nolan, 1992). Evidence from studies which also obtained clinical data on respondents suggests a high degree of agreement with such self-reports.

Table 2 *Chronic Physical Illness by Age and Social Class, Ireland 1987*

Age range	social class					
	higher professional	lower professional	other non-manual	skilled manual	semi-skilled manual	unskilled manual
	% reporting chronic illness					
15–34	5.1	2.9	5.3	9.2	7.9	10.0
35–44	5.6	5.8	9.4	11.2	15.4	12.3
45–54	11.0	13.0	16.7	19.2	23.5	27.0
55–64	23.5	22.0	28.2	28.9	32.6	44.7
65 and over	21.8	33.6	30.8	37.6	36.3	33.4
all	10.5	10.5	13.9	17.0	19.0	24.6

Many of those with serious long-standing illnesses will give their current labour force status as ill or disabled rather than unemployed, so the relationship with current unemployment is problematic. Nonetheless, those who are currently unemployed in the ESRI sample were more likely to report a long-standing illness than those in work, controlling for age. (For example, for those aged between 35 and 44, 16% of those currently unemployed, but only 5% of employees, reported such an illness). It is, however, more the relationship between unemployment and ill-health over time which is the nub of the issue. The ESRI survey also reveals that those who had experienced unemployment in their careers were more likely to have also spent time away from work because of illness than those who had not experienced unemployment. Similarly, a high proportion of those who were away from work due to illness or disability at the time of the survey had also experienced unemployment during their careers.

The factors producing the observed relationship between physical ill-health and socio-economic background, and between ill-health and unemployment in particular, are complex and difficult to disentangle. The poverty and deprivation often associated with membership of lower socio-economic groups can have direct effects through for example poor nutrition and housing conditions. Behavioural factors which may increase risk of particular illnesses are also more prevalent in lower socio-economic groups, and certain occupations may involve exposure to specific risks. As far as unemployment is concerned, it is suggested that the psychological stresses involved may also play an important role in increasing vulnerability to physical illnesses. It is extremely difficult, with the types of data usually available, to distinguish the role of different factors, or to isolate the impact of unemployment per se from that of the broader socio-economic background from which those experiencing unemployment generally come.

Unemployment and Psychological Distress

A variety of studies employing rather different methodological approaches converge in establishing the causal impact of unemployment on psychological distress. In the ESRI survey conducted in 1987, the measure of psychological distress employed the General Health Questionnaire (GHQ) in its 12-item format. (Whelan *et al.*, 1991; Whelan, 1992 and 1994). The GHQ was designed by Goldberg (1972) as a screening test for detecting minor psychiatric disorders in the community. The items included in the measure are designed to give information about the respondent's current mental state. It is neither a measure of long-standing attributes of personality, nor an assessment of the likelihood of falling ill in the near future (Goldberg, 1972). It is most definitely not, however, a mere complaints inventory. It consists only of items that have been chosen from a substantial battery of items shown to discriminate between groups of respondents in terms of their likelihood of being assessed as non-psychotic psychiatric cases.

If the results of a set of GHQ scores are compared with an independent psychiatric assessment, it is possible to state the number of symptoms at which the probability that an individual will be thought to be a psychiatric case exceeds one half. In the case of the twelve-item version, the threshold score is 2 and all respondents scoring above this level will be classified as suffering from psychological distress. Since the conclusions we wish to draw remain true irrespective of whether a dichotomous or continuous measure is employed, we will present our results in terms of the former, not just because of their intrinsic interest but also because it facilitates the communication of our most important results.

Using the GHQ measure we find that, as can be seen from Figure 1, just over *one in three* of the unemployed come above the psychological distress threshold compared to *one in fourteen* of employees. The differentials between these groups on selected individual items are documented in Figure 2. Only departures from usual functioning are scored as pathological and not responses such as 'no more than usual'. Despite this, almost 36% of unemployed men give a response in the pathological category to the question regarding feeling unhappy and depressed. Over 20% or more *in each case* indicate that they:

    (i)   felt they couldn't overcome their difficulties;
   (ii)   lost much sleep over worry;
 (iii)   felt constantly under strain;
 (iv)   have been losing confidence in themselves.

The disparities between the unemployed and the employees on such items range from 2 to 1 to 4 to 1. On perhaps the most extreme negative item in the set – 'been thinking of yourself as a worthless person' – the level of

Figure 1: *Percentage with scores above the general health questionnaire threshold: a comparison of unemployed and employees*

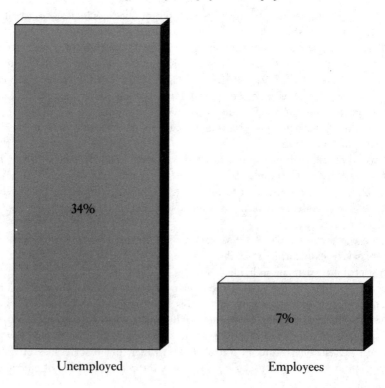

34%

7%

Unemployed   Employees

Figure 2: *A comparison of the level of negative response on
selected general health questionnaire items for unemployed and employees*

Been feeling unhappy and depressed

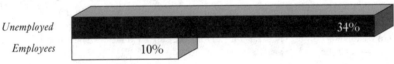

Unemployed   34%

Employees   10%

Been unable to face up to your problems

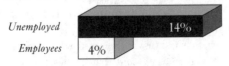

Unemployed   14%

Employees   4%

Lost much sleep over worry

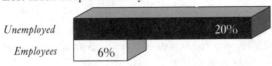

Unemployed   20%

Employees   6%

Felt that you are not playing a useful part in things

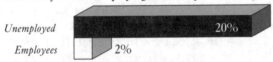

Unemployed   20%

Employees   2%

Been thinking of yourself as a worthless person

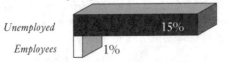

Unemployed   15%

Employees   1%

pathological response is lower for the unemployed than on the other negative
items, i.e., 14%. The differential, however, between the unemployed and
employees of 17 to 1 is the highest on any of the items.

Length of Unemployment

The concept of stages of unemployment which emerged in the literature of
the 1930s has become a basic concept in accounts of the psychological effects
of unemployment. Eisenberg and Lazarfeld (1938: 378) concluded:

> We find that all writers who have described the course of unemployment seem to agree on the following points: first there is shock, which is followed by an active hunt for a job, during which the individual is still optimistic and unresigned; he still maintains an unbroken attitude.
>
> Second, when all efforts fail, the individual becomes pessimistic, anxious and suffers active distress: this is the most crucial state of all. And third the individual becomes fatalistic and adapts himself to his new state but with a narrower scope. He now has a broken attitude.

Studies relating length of unemployment to mental health, however, have been far from consistent. Jackson and Warr (1984) suggest that the failure of early studies to find a relationship may have been due to the fact that the age range of respondents or the length of unemployment studies were too restricted. More recent studies suggest that the newly unemployed experience a deterioration in psychological health within weeks and that by three months this has become worse, but it then remains stable for long periods and might even improve (Fryer and Payne, 1986).

Our own results, which are set out in Figure 3, show little difference between those employed for less than a year and those unemployed more than one year. These results are consistent with the findings in the literature. However, this contrast conceals some interesting differences. If we exclude those seeking their first job and those on State training schemes, we find that levels of mental decline beyond the second year of unemployment with the level of psychological distress increasing from 37% above the threshold for those unemployed for less than two years to 43% for those between two to three years, and to 54% for those above between three to four years; at this point it drops dramatically to 25% for those unemployed more than four years. With the exception of this final result, our findings are consistent with the hypothesis of a gradual decline in psychological well-being.

The explanation of this latter finding requires that we turn our attention to the relationship between unemployment and poverty. It is important to keep in mind, as Kelvin and Jarrett (1985: 26) stress that:

> The description of stages does not itself provide an explanation of the effects of unemployment: at most it merely provides the first step towards it, and that only if the description is sufficiently accurate.

What is necessary, they argue, is to isolate the factors which determine the transition between stages and developments within them. Despite the attention devoted to stages, Kelvin and Jarrett (1985: 19–30) note that there have been very few attempts to trace the interaction of the economic and psychological effects of unemployment and to move beyond description to examine the systematic relationship between increasing poverty and changing reactions to unemployment.

Figure 3: *Percentage above general health questionnaire*
threshold score by length of unemployment

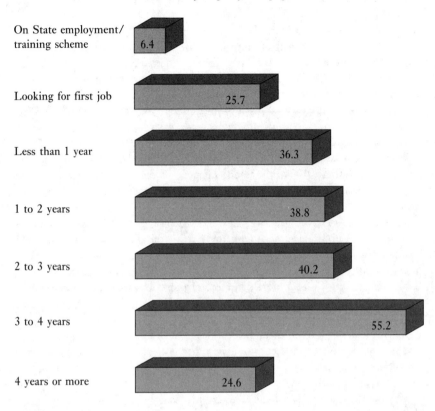

On State employment/
training scheme — 6.4

Looking for first job — 25.7

Less than 1 year — 36.3

1 to 2 years — 38.8

2 to 3 years — 40.2

3 to 4 years — 55.2

4 years or more — 24.6

Again, if we exclude those seeking their first job and those on State schemes, we find that the percentage falling below our poverty line rises steadily with length of unemployment. This result makes our previous finding regarding the relatively low levels of distress displayed by those unemployed for more than four years even more perplexing. This finding tends to undermine an explanation of the 'deviant' result in terms of participation in the 'black economy'. An alternative explanation could be offered in terms of coping adjustments. Warr and Jackson identify two particularly important mechanisms of adaptation to a new role and reduced commitment to finding a new job. This interpretation takes into account the fact that the initial period of unemployment may be a particularly traumatic time. Gradually adaptation may take place.

Daily and weekly routines become established, expenditure limits become clarified and behaviour may be shaped to avoid threats from new situations or other people (Warr and Jackson, 1985: 805).

A further adjustment arises from the calculation that the probability of obtaining paid work is low, with a consequent reduction in employment commitment and job seeking.

Set against such possibilities is the increased probability of poverty. It seems doubtful to us, in view of the latter, that such coping strategies could account for the results we have observed. It is necessary, therefore, to consider a further possibility raised by Warr and Jackson (1985: 806) that the type of response alternative employed in our measure of psychological distress may lead to an underestimation of levels of distress of those in long-term unemployment. The GHQ may miss chronic disorders because it asks respondents for an assessment of symptoms in terms of categories such as 'same as usual'. This seems to occur less than might be expected on theoretical grounds because people cling rather stubbornly to the concept of their 'usual self'. It seems plausible, though, that those unemployed for more than five years may have great difficulty in preserving such a concept.

It is necessary to emphasise, however, that although length of unemployment does produce some interesting effects, the differences are relatively modest. Such differences are much less important than the fact of being unemployed (Fryer and Payne, 1986: 253). Similarly, previous unemployment has a weak effect. Thus, a mere 2% more of those who had been unemployed in the past twelve months were above the GHQ case threshold than those who were at work and had never been unemployed. In relation to the impact of unemployment on physical health, the available evidence suggests that one should avoid an undue emphasis on current spell of unemployment since it diverts attention away from the accumulation of disadvantages over time. With mental health, on the other hand, it does appear that the current employment situation is critical. This finding is consistent with the evidence that re-employment leads very rapidly to dramatic improvements in mental health.

Unemployment, Poverty and Psychological Distress

In surveying the current literature on the psychological distress, a compelling case can be made that its most striking feature is the remarkable lack of emphasis on poverty. A great deal of the literature relating to the impact of unemployment on mental health has operated from a perspective that views levels of distress as influenced by life events, with unemployment constituting one such crucial life event.

The earlier studies espoused the idea that a straightforward numerical accumulation of experienced life events predisposes to illness. Underlying this approach is the assumption that events lead to stress because the organism is fundamentally intolerant of change, an assumption which was rooted in the pioneering laboratory studies. The natural state of the organism was seen as one of equilibrium.

Social scientists have increasingly questioned the notion that change *per se* is damaging. They have moved beyond notions relating to the number of events and the magnitude of change in terms of degree of adjustment and have focused attention on issues relating to the quality of events – desirability, degree of control, whether or not they are scheduled or unscheduled (Pearlin *et al.*, 1981).

Unemployment is clearly an event which is predominantly undesirable, uncontrolled and unscheduled. It has generally been labelled an acute stressor and fits readily within the stressful life change approach. Stress, however, can follow both from change in the environment and lack of change (Wheaton, 1980). It is useful to distinguish between acute stressors and chronic stressors. Chronic stress arises from the dogged, slow-to-change, problems of daily life, when pressures from the environment exceed the coping capacity of the person. The two types of stress converge when life changes have an impact by increasing the number and level of day-to-day life strains. The impact on emotional well-being in such cases arises, not from change itself, but from change that leads to hardship in basic enduring economic and social circumstances. The most striking example of this process is when unemployment leads to economic hardship and social isolation both for individuals and their family (Pearlin *et al.*, 1981). Kelvin and Jarrett (1985: 18) note that while those concerned with the psychology of work have long stressed that work provides much more than merely money; those concerned with unemployment need to stress that to be unemployed is frequently to be poor.

When we look at the relationship between poverty and mental health in the Irish case, using a poverty line which combines information on income and life-style, we find that one in three of the poor come above the psychological distress threshold compared to one in eight of the non-poor (Callan *et al.*, 1994).

The issue of the relative importance of unemployment and poverty must, to some extent, be an artificial one since unemployment is one of the major causes of poverty. The evidence, though, is clearly relevant to the issue of the relative significance of manifest and latent functions of employment. Jahoda (1981, 1982) argues that over and above the provision of financial rewards, employment serves a variety of latent functions by embedding the individual in a web of social relations. Our empirical analysis does indeed show that unemployment has a significant effect even among the non-poor, with those who are unemployed being five times more likely to come above the psychological threshold than those who are at work or retired. However, our results clearly indicate that the impact of unemployment is mediated, to a significant extent, by exposure to poverty. The cumulative impact of unemployment and poverty is illustrated by the fact that while less than one in fourteen of those at work or retired and non-poor exhibited mental health problems, the figure rose to well over four out of ten for those who suffer both poverty and unemployment.

References

Brenner, M.H. (1979) Unemployment and health, *Lancet*, 874–5.
Brenner, M.H. (1983) Mortality and economic instability: detailed analyses for Britain and comparative analyses for selected industrialised countries, *International Journal of Health Services*, 13: 563–620.
Eisenberg, P. and P. Lazarfeld (1938) The psychological effects of unemployment, *Psychological Bulletin*, 35: 358–90.
Fox A., P. Goldblatt and D. Jones (1985) Social class mortality differentials: artefact selection or life circumstances in: R. Wilkinson (ed.) *Class and Health*. London: Tavistock.
Fryer, D. (1992) Psychological or material deprivation? in E. McLaughlin (ed.) *Understanding Unemployment: new perspectives on Active Labour Market Policies*. London: Routledge.
Fryer, D. and R. Payne (1986) Being unemployed: a review of the literature on the psychological experience of unemployment, in: C. Cooper and I. Robertson (eds) *International Review of International and Organisational Psychology*.
Goldberg, P. (1972) *On the Detection of Psychiatric Illness by Questionnaire*. London: Oxford University Press.
Goldblatt, P. (1989) Mortality by social class 1971–85, *Population Trends*, 56.
Jackson, P.R. and P.B. Warr (1984) Unemployment and psychological ill-health: the moderating role of duration and age, *Psychological Medicine*, 14: 605–14.
Jahoda, M. (1981) Work, employment and unemployment: values, theories and approaches in social research, *American Psychologist*, 36: 181–91.
Jahoda, M. (1982) *Employment and Unemployment: A Social-Psychological Analysis*, Cambridge: Cambridge University Press.
Kelvin, P. and T. Jarrett (1985) *Unemployment: Its Social Psychological Effects*. Cambridge: Cambridge University Press.
Moser, K., A. Fox and D. Jones (1984) Unemployment and mortality in the OPCS longitudinal survey, *Lancet*, 8 December: 1342–9.
Nolan, B. (1990) Social economic mortality differentials in Ireland, *Economic and Social Review*, 21 (2): 193–208.
Nolan, B. (1992) Poverty and health inequalities, in: T. Callan and B. Nolan (eds) *Poverty in Ireland*. Dublin: Gill & Macmillan.
Nolan, B. And T. Callan (eds) (1994) *Poverty and Policy in Ireland*, Dublin: Gill & Macmillan.
Pearlin, L., E. Menaghan, M. Lieberman and J.T. Mullan (1981) The stress process, *Journal of Health and Social Behaviour*, 22: 3337–51
Smith, R. (1987) *Unemployment and Health: A Disaster and a Challenge*. Oxford: Oxford University Press.
Warr, P.B. (1987) *Work, Unemployment and Mental Health*. Oxford: Clarendon Press.
Warr, P.B. and P. Jackson (1985) Men without jobs: some correlates of age and length of unemployment, *Journal of Occupational Psychology*, 57 (1): 77–86.

Warr, P.B. and P. Jackson (1985) Factors influencing the psychological impact of prolonged unemployment and of re-employment, *Psychological Medicine*, 15: 795–817.

Wheaton, B. (1980) The sociogenesis of psychological disorder: an attributional theory, *Journal of Health and Social Behaviour*, 21: 100–24.

Whelan, C.T., D.F. Hannan and S. Creighton (1991) Unemployment, poverty and psychological distress, *General Research Series*, No. 150, Dublin: Economic and Social Research Institute.

Whelan, C.T. (1992) The role of income, life-style deprivation and financial strain in mediating the impact of unemployment of psychological distress: evidence from the Republic of Ireland, *Journal of Occupational and Organisational Psychology*, 64: 331–44.

Whelan, C.T. (1994) Social class, unemployment, psychological distress, *European Sociological Review*, 10 (1): 49–62.

Section 3

HEALTH ISSUES AND LIFE COURSE

7

The Medicalisation of Childbearing Norms: Encounters Between Unmarried Pregnant Women and Medical Personnel in an Irish Context

Abbey Hyde

Introduction

This chapter is based on the accounts of a sample of unmarried pregnant women and focuses on medical interest in the social organisation of the women's reproductive practices. It is argued that medical jurisdiction can stretch beyond physiological aspects of pregnancy to concerns with normative social standards, whereby wider social discourses on the timing and context of childbearing in women's lives are brought to bear during medical encounters. Medicine can lay claim to this 'social' aspect of women's lives through appeals to holism and 'social health'; however, the notion of social health is contentious in that medicine's cues to problematise a pregnancy in a social sense are rooted in wider discourses on normality. Medicine's assessment of a socially 'questionable' pregnancy in turn contributes to the construction of normative boundaries for childbearing.

While medicine's potential to operate as an institution of social control is well established within medical sociology (Zola, 1972; Foucault, 1973; Illich, 1976; Armstrong, 1993, 1995a, 1995b) and public health medicine (Skrabanek, 1994), feminist sociologists in particular have elucidated the medical appropriation of childbirth, which was previously constructed as a natural process (Oakley, 1980; Murphy-Lawless 1988a, 1988b; Lupton, 1994). The medical takeover of physiological aspects of childbirth is one issue; a second – and centrally important for this paper – is at least some medical practitioners' use of moral judgements on the social circumstances of pregnancy, and the impact these have on the nature of medical interactions.

'Unmarried mothers' have long been institutionalised and categorised by the medical profession for transgressions of societal norms. Murphy-Lawless's

(1988c) historical analysis of male medical midwives (early obstetricians) in the Rotunda Hospital in the last century elucidates the mediation of moral and physiological boundaries in relation to non-marital mothers in the contemporary period. Post-natal puerperal fever suffered by unmarried women was causally linked to the distress of 'seduction' and their non-marital status (Murphy-Lawless, 1988c). More recently, Sally Macintyre (1977) in a Scottish study found that medical practitioners constituted categories of women based on the latter's sexual histories and behaviour and used these to make 'medical' decisions (for example, whether or not to sanction an abortion). Macintyre (1991) also noted how women's marital status influenced the medical interpretation of post-natal depression; for married women, this was normalised, while for single women it was perceived in terms of ambivalence towards the infant. Finlay and Shaw (1993) have also identified tension between medical and scientific issues on the one hand, and moral issues on the other, in the arguments proposed by the Department of Public Health Medicine in Northern Ireland for the initiation of a Brook Centre in Belfast to deal with the 'problem' of teenage pregnancy.

It is argued here that the recent emphasis on 'holistic medicine' (Armstrong, 1995a) serves to legitimate medicine's concern with psycho-social areas of childbirth, and can operate as a mechanism of social control in distinguishing problematic from acceptable pregnancies. As well as furnishing further evidence to support the broad notion that at least some physicians extend their intervention into delimiting socially approved reproductive arrangements, this paper explores the place of 'holism' in the care of pregnant women. It is argued that what a number of participants in this study reported was a kind of 'paternalistic holism' whereby obstetricians assessed women's health status and acted according to normative dictates, with the impact of problematising pregnancies without adequately considering participants' versions of their circumstances.

Firstly, the methodological stance of the study will be outlined. This will be followed by data that buttress the argument that non-marital motherhood continues to be problematised by medical personnel.

Methodological Stance

Fifty-one study participants were selected from the Out-Patient Clinic of a large maternity hospital in Dublin to which access was successfully gained via the medical and midwifery directors. Inclusion criteria were that potential partakers would not be married to the father of the foetus and be first-time expectant mothers. The age range of participants was 16 to 36 years with 12 of the women under 20 years at the time of the birth. Informed consent was obtained and anonymity guaranteed. Those who assented to partake were informed of their freedom to withdraw from the study at any time. Ninety women were invited to participate of whom 51 were eventually interviewed.[1]

In-depth semi-structured interviews were held on two separate occasions: firstly in the third trimester of pregnancy, and secondly, in almost all cases, between weeks six and eight after the birth. The interviews were conducted from mid-1992 to late 1993. Since the present paper is concerned with medical encounters during the pregnancy, accounts presented here are from the first interviews.

The study adopted a qualitative approach from a pluralist feminist standpoint position in order to centralise participants' experiences in medical encounters. The standpoint position, first proposed within feminist thought by writers such as Hartsock (1983, 1987), Rose (1983, 1986), and Smith (1979, 1987), contends that the dominance of conceptual schemes rooted in male perspectives of the social world has meant partiality and distortion in understanding events. Such biases may only be amended, it deems, by manifesting an understanding of the world from the perspective of women's activities (Harding, 1989). More recently, a *pluralist* standpoint position has been advanced (Gelsthorpe, 1992) in response to criticisms directed at earlier universal models of patriarchy that paid insufficient attention to differences in women's experiences arising from variations in class, race, sexual identity and so forth. The notion of plurality acknowledges that while women have a particular perspective as women, their characteristics and situations vary, resulting in a variety of 'uniquely valid insights' (Gelsthorpe, 1992: 215).

A grounded theory style of analysis (Glaser and Strauss, 1967; Glaser, 1978, 1992; Strauss, 1987; Strauss and Corbin, 1990, 1994) was used to code data qualitatively, although this strategy was utilised selectively. As data collection progressed, questions about topics became increasingly focused around theoretically pertinent issues and concepts. A constant comparative method was employed, whereby like items of data were clustered and later theorised. In contrast to quantitative research where support for an argument is based primarily (and sometimes solely) on *enumerating* the empirical support for a theoretical position, in qualitative analyses, along with empirical breadth, the quality of data and its conceptual relevance is considered important (Dey, 1993).[2]

Medical Encounters

Three issues reported by participants concerning medical encounters will be singled out for conceptual purposes, although these overlapped considerably. The areas are: 1. Medical practitioners introducing the notion of adoption; 2. Participants being pressurised to see the social worker; 3. The questioning of participants about social arrangements for childcare or their capacity to parent.

Medical practitioners introducing the notion of adoption

Adoption has long been associated with unwanted pregnancies, and to suggest adoption to a pregnant woman is to raise questions about the acceptability of the pregnancy. A considerable number of women reported that the issue of adoption was raised at the hospital in various interactions with professionals, including medical doctors. Some women were overtly dissatisfied with adoption being raised, especially as in Angela's case below, where the issue was broached repetitively:

> Angela: The first time I went to the hospital I went to the public ward, the time I met you . . . Every single comment was the fact that I wasn't married. Every single one of them. It was, 'Are you keeping the baby?'
>
> Interviewer: Who was it that asked you that?
>
> Angela: The nurse that gave me the blood test and then the doctor said the same thing to me, 'Are you keeping the baby?'
>
> . . . The doctor that saw me in the public clinic, I didn't really like. I mean I'm not like, paranoid, but he did have sort of a patronising attitude, and it did irritate me when he said that, 'Are you keeping the baby?' because it was written down. I felt like saying, 'Can you not read?' (32-year-old engineer.)

Some women had no doubt that the line of enquiry was directly related to their single status, or, as in Iris's case, their age, in so far as married women would not experience the same questions:

> Iris: They asked me [at the hospital] would I think of adoption.
>
> Interviewer: How did you feel about that kind of questioning?
>
> Iris: Nearly died. I thought it was just because I was young. And you know the way they ask you if you're single, married or divorced or something. I said I was single, and em, he asked me would I be into adoption, would I think about it, and I knew it was a question he wouldn't ask a married person or an older person . . .
> . . . I felt a bit intimidated, like [inaudible].   (21-year-old office clerk.)

A number of women who recalled being asked about the issue of adoption accepted such questioning, suggesting their internalisation of wider social norms around childbearing:

> Interviewer: Did he ask you anything about the baby?
>
> Kim: Yeah, he asked me if I was going to keep the baby, and I said 'yeah', and that was it.
>
> Interviewer: How did you feel about being asked?
>
> Kim: I didn't mind. It didn't bother me. I was expecting to be asked that.
>   (21-year-old cleaner.)

Beyond the hospital, some women had encounters with General Practitioners (GP) during the pregnancy and while most GPs did not discuss pregnancy-outcome options with the women, a small number of participants did recall episodes where the issue of adoption was raised. In Trish's case, following a discussion on abortion, her GP attempted to propel her towards a decision to place the baby for adoption:

> Trish: I was just thinking, 'What am I going to do?' and I did think of having an abortion. I was just so messed up, and he [the GP] was talking to me against [pause], but he wasn't – he was saying like what it could do to you if I did . . . and he was saying that he wouldn't pressure me either way – that it was my decision at the end of the day but he just wanted me to know that [pause], he was telling me about different cases that he had experienced and how they were finding it even after years – that you think everything is wonderful but that it can come back and hit you. . .
>
> . . . He then said about adoption. He annoyed me, 'cause he kept going on about it. He was saying, 'You don't realise the responsibilities', and bla, bla, bla. And I'm going 'Jesus, like, I have thought'. . .   (22-year-old receptionist.)

A number of women in Macintyre's (1977) study resented their GPs suggesting pregnancy outcomes other than those they had already intended to pursue, because this had inferences for the kind of definition of the situation that was negotiated in the encounter. A number of participants in the present study similarly took exception to propositions of alternatives from medical professionals. This was because any proposal of alternatives would frame their circumstances as aberrant by undermining the perceived unquestionable assumption that the baby was being raised by its natural parent or parents, as would occur in any 'normal' situation, even if the participant was unmarried and/or unpartnered.

Participants being pressurised to see the social worker

It would seem to be a positive and useful practice to offer a social work service to those who might require public assistance during their pregnancies. However, aside from situations where the practice is for all patients to be informed that a social work service is available to them, the offer of a social work service on a selective basis is to construe particular pregnancies as more potentially problematic than others. The practice at the hospital where participants were selected was to identify all unmarried women as candidates for at least one interview with the social worker. Those who circumvented the social worker on their first visit were identified by a sticker placed on their case notes. A number of women slipped through the net, and some who did not voluntarily accept the offer to see the social worker were coerced into doing so by the medical consultant. To be accompanied by a medical escort (the consultant) to the Social Work Department after a medical check-up was by no means uncommon among those women who managed to elude the social workers on earlier visits:

> Janet: So the next time I went to the hospital then, I got this doctor who was really cranky. He was going on about smoking . . . Then he examined me. He didn't tell me anything. That was it, like, it was two minutes. So then he says, 'Come with me.' Walked out of the room, marched me down to the social worker.

> Interviewer: How did you feel about that?

> Janet: I didn't know where I was going or what he was doing, and I was, I was looking at him and he had a hold of the chart. I thought he was just bringing me into reception or something. And we walked by reception, so I just kept on following him. I was a bit taken aback you know kind of and he said to me, 'Sit down there', he said, 'The social worker will be with you in a minute.' I said, 'Hold on a minute. . .' and he walked off.

> Interviewer: How did you feel about that?

> Janet: I was still stunned after what he was after saying to me in the room about the smoking, you know, even though I know he's right about smoking. It was just his attitude, the way he was actually speaking to me, you know. . . So em, the social worker came along and eh, she brought me into the room and I said, 'Why do I have to see you? Why do I have to see a social worker? And she said, 'We just make a point of seeing unmarried mothers, or people who are separated.' I said, 'I'm fine, I don't want to see a social worker,' and she said, 'Well, we'll just check you out anyway.' And I was thinking, like, I could be married and have problems and they wouldn't make a point of seeing me, you know.   (23-year-old waitress.)

> Pauline: I never realised you have to see the social worker. The student midwife who came in to me, she said, 'Oh you'll have to see the social worker.' She said, 'You can make an appointment today and come in another day.' But he [doctor] said to me, 'While you're here, I'll bring you to the social worker.' So, he just brought me up, and like you were going out of the room and around by all the different places. I was conscious of that and even [partner] was too cause he followed me, and he goes, 'What's wrong?' And I said 'Nothing'. Like people waiting hadn't got an idea where I was going but I had. But even [partner] didn't know. . .

> . . . I should have said something, but I didn't.   (20-year-old secretary.)

While a number of women, as the examples above suggest, were most unhappy about being ushered to the social worker in such a manner, others, amazingly, accepted this situation without question:

> Darina: They asked me did I go to the social worker and I said no, cause I didn't know what I had to see her for. Then on the second visit there was a sticker on me chart, 'Patient must see social worker on next visit.' But the doctor marched me down on me last visit [laughs].

Interviewer: How did you feel about that?

Darina: It didn't bother me. . .

(21-year-old, unemployed.)

Kim: . . . I was walked down to the social worker by the doctor.

Interviewer: Were you?

Kim: That didn't really bother me. There was a note on me chart, 'Go see social worker'. I meant to go the first time but didn't. The thoughts of it!

(21-year-old cleaner.)

The Questioning of Participants' Arrangements for Childcare or Capacity to Parent

Some participants were questioned by medical practitioners about their plans for childcare, insinuating that their social circumstances for childrearing were deemed by medical professionals to be possibly sub-standard, or at least questionable:

Penny: The first visit I went to [the hospital] I thought the doctor was very rude because I wasn't married, and he was asking me was I keeping the baby, and was I going back to work, and I said, 'Yeah,' and he asked me who I was going to get to mind the baby, which put me off. It was none of his business anyway. I felt it was nothing to do with him whether I'd go back to work or who'd mind the baby. (24-year-old receptionist.)

Interviewer: How was the visit to the doctor?

Pauline: . . . and the first thing he said to me was – he looked at me chart and he said, 'Miss [her name]', and I said, 'Yes', And he said, 'Do you plan on keeping this child?' in a real stern voice. And I said, 'Oh my God, what other way is he going to scrutinise me, you know.' And I said, 'Yes', and he said, 'Well how do you plan on keeping this child?' 'Oh my God!' I said. And I said, 'With the help of me mam and me mam's friend.' (20-year-old secretary.)

An additional participant's capacity to meet the demands of motherhood was questioned by her GP:

Trish: And I just couldn't understand why he kept going on at me like [to consider adoption], when I was saying I don't want it. And he's going, 'You don't realise the responsibilities.' And then my mother was down for something else and he said to her to talk to me 'cause 'I don't think she [participant] realises what's involved.' (22-year-old receptionist.)

In the absence of a group of married women with which to compare the medical encounters of unmarried women, one can only speculate as to the interactions married women might experience; however, it would seem most unlikely that married women would be subjected to the kind of questioning explored above.

It was notable that those women who were most dissatisfied about an issue being made about their single status tended to be among the better educated of those attending the public clinic. Women from the highest socio-economic groups attended the semi-private clinic, and these reportedly did not experience a sense of problematisation of the pregnancy by the medical profession to the same extent.

Discussion

The notion that medical involvement in non-marital pregnancies frequently surpassed a focus on the physio-medical component was supported by data in relation to the three areas presented above: physicians interposing the issue of adoption during the medical encounter; participants' being pressurised (and in some cases compelled) to visit the social worker; and medical practitioners enquiring about participants' childcare plans or potential to parent adequately. Medicine's extension beyond physio-medical aspects of childbirth will be explored here in relation to the concept of holism, and the difficulties associated with 'social health' when this blurs with the notion of social control.

Although it is not known whether the physicians referred to above identified with a holistic agenda in extending beyond strictly 'medical' concerns (in its narrow sense), medicine might legitimately argue that any accusations of surveillance or social control place it in a difficult position. Holistic care implies an appreciation of the multiple aspects of the human person, including physical, social, psychological and spiritual. In showing no interest in social aspects of the pregnancy, physicians might be accused of reverting to 'reductionist' medicine (Armstrong, 1995a: 45) with concern only for the individual (physical) parts of the person. In practising some notion of holistic medicine by encompassing 'social health' they might be censured for social surveillance.

The style of holistic care adopted in medical encounters presented in this paper could be coined 'paternalistic holism' in so far as, in the unequal relations between practitioners and participants, women were seen to be unable to decide what was in their own interest (for example, to visit the social worker), so physicians imposed this practice on women for their own good. This could then be justified on the grounds of care and concern with social health, for example – a need to ensure that unmarried women were aware of their social and welfare rights. However noble the intentions of medical practitioners were in this respect, the difficulties with this practice are obvious. It reinforces women's passivity, and takes the issue of choice and agency out of their hands. Furthermore, dominance is displayed by medical professionals in defining appropriate circumstances for childbearing, that is, medical professionals have a standard for how social reproduction should be organised (a family unit with two married parents).

A solution oft-referred to in the 'caring' literature is to use a non-judgmental approach when assessing a person's health status. One possibility is that during the midwives' assessment, all pregnant women irrespective of marital status could be asked the same questions about their perceptions of the pregnancy, and those who view their own pregnancy ambiguously would then be offered social work services. However, this generalised approach might contravene to some extent the notion of individualised care often associated with holistic practice (Department of Health and Social Welfare, 1984). Aside from this, the reality of using an entirely 'non-judgmental' approach in assessing social health is questionable given that some judgement has been made even to raise issues that might suggest that the status of a pregnancy was equivocal. The yardstick for such judgement is most likely to be relativism, with what is considered to be 'normal' social health getting its cues from wider society, and in turn contributing to them. 'Social health' is poorly defined in the literature, opening up the possibility that, in practice, anti-social behaviour or actions that are at variance with established rules of conduct will be treated as pathological.

The extent of medicine's power in creating the boundaries of 'normality' in the social organisation of reproduction or in simply reinforcing normative discourses emanating elsewhere is open to question. An analysis of a variety of Irish newspapers[3] would seem to suggest that dominant discourses expressing disquiet about non-marital motherhood are rooted in economics (welfare dependence) rather than in medical concerns, or religion as was previously the case; however medical concerns cannot be dismissed easily as these feature in apprehensions expressed about the psychological impact of absent fathers and concomitant anti-social behaviour of children from fatherless families. Whether medicine, economics, religion, some other realm, or a variety of these, is the driving force in the construction of discourses on the social regulation of reproduction, it is clear from data presented here that, whether it intended it or not, medicine at least plays a part in the maintenance of social order around social arrangements for childbearing.

Practices which maintain social order were evident in each category of data presented. Promoting adoption supports the two-heterosexual-parent family and reduces the possibility of deviant family formations. Insisting on social work contact exposes the client to social work advice, which tends to promote dual parenting, contact with the putative father where the relationship had ended, or adoption (Hyde, 1996). It also implicitly reminds the client that non-marital childbearing is not fully acceptable, and this may act as a deterrent (along with other messages they receive) to future non-marital pregnancies. Questioning women on their childcare plans and/or competence at mothering suggests that fathers are necessary to adequate childcare; ironically, while it must be acknowledged that some fathers take equal responsibility for childcare, most empirical studies suggest that fathers do not engage in day-to-day childcare to anything like the same extent as mothers

(Croghan, 1991; Richardson, 1993; Market Research Bureau of Ireland, 1992; Kiely, 1995; O'Connor, 1995). However, as McKee (1982: 129) notes, irrespective of their level of practical involvement, men are seen to offer the 'spirit' of support to wives and the 'moral context' for childcare.

This paper has provided new evidence to support the notion that some medical practitioners make value judgements about pregnancies that threaten social order, and that these judgements mediate medical encounters. At a theoretical level, the issue of holism and its potential for social control were considered in light of the data. Holistic medicine has the potential to legitimate what might previously have been deemed to be beyond the confines of medicine. It is argued that what women in some encounters experienced was 'paternalistic holism' where physicians seemed to determine what was in their best interests without always involving them in the decision. Medical practitioners' constructions of non-marital pregnancies tended to rest easily with society's dominant (albeit challenged) values in relation to the social organisation of reproduction.

Notes

[1] Since data collection in this study was confined to interviews with pregnant women, the analysis is not concerned with presenting any kind of 'objective reality' of medical encounters (even if this could ever be achieved). Rather it endeavours to understand women's subjective experiences of such encounters. The interpretation of data is based on comprehending participants' constructions of such interactions, and locating these within wider social processes.

[2] Dey (1993: 225) notes how qualitative data is characteristically uneven in quality, which justifies 'giving extra salience to part of the data in conceptual terms even if this is out of proportion to its empirical scope'. Nonetheless, the weight of evidence in support of a theoretical position is important, and an assessment of this is facilitated by looking for, not just corroborating evidence, but also inconsistent and contradictory accounts (Dey, 1993). While aspects of data in support of the overall argument being presented in this paper pertain to 'some' or a 'considerable proportion' of women, this, at least in part, reflects the unevenness of qualitative data referred to by Dey (1993). While there is no suggestion that the encounters analysed in this paper represent all medical encounters experienced by study participants, the overall picture reveals an empirical expanse much greater than a few isolated cases.

[3] Although the analysis of Irish newspapers was rather crude, articles or letters from a wide variety of newspapers were included. These newspapers were:

Irish Independent, 26/03/87; 23/05/87; 23/08/87; 10/09/87; 10/02/88; 30/11/88; 13/03/89; 02/05/89; 25/05/89; 14/06/89; 10/11/89; 01/10/90; 13/11/91; 01/05/92; 6/05/92; 13/06/92; 03/09/93; 09/09/93.

Irish Press, 23/05/87; 10/09/88; 25/01/92.

The Irish Times, 16/02/72; 17/02/72; 18/02/72; 09/05/87; 10/09/87; 05/11/87; 28/12/87; 26/07/88; 28/01/89; 25/05/89; 26/07/90; 25/02/92; 24/04/93; 13/10/93; 19/10/93; 04/03/94; 07/03/94; 27/05/94; 09/11/94; 13/12/94.

Sunday Independent, 20/07/87.

Sunday Tribune, 16/04/89; 31/10/93.

The Star, 13/04/89; 23/09/92; 28/09/93.

References

Armstrong, D. (1993) From clinical gaze to regime of total health, in: A. Beattie, M. Gott, L. Jones and M. Sidell (eds), *Health and Well-being: A Reader*. Basingstoke: Macmillan: 55–67.

Armstrong, D. (1995a) The problem of the whole-person in holistic medicine, in: B. Davey, A. Gray, and C. Seale (eds) *Health and Disease: A Reader* (2nd edition). Buckingham: Open University Press: 45–9

Armstrong, D. (1995b) The rise of surveillance medicine, *Sociology of Health and Illness*, 17 (3): 393–404.

Croghan, R. (1991) First-time mothers' accounts of inequality in the division of labour, *Feminism and Psychology*, 1 (2): 221–46.

Department of Health and Social Welfare (1984) *A Systematic Approach to Nursing Care: An Introduction*. Milton Keynes: Open University.

Dey, I. (1993) *Qualitative Data Analysis*. London: Routledge.

Finlay, A. and N. Shaw (1993) Teenage pregnancy and the controversy surrounding Brook in Belfast, *Critical Public Health*, 4 (2): 24–30.

Foucault, M. (1973) *The Birth of the Clinic: An Archaeology of Medical Perception*. London: Tavistock.

Gelsthorpe, L. (1992) Response to Martin Hammersley's paper, 'On feminist methodology', *Sociology*, 26 (2): 213–18.

Glaser, B. (1978) *Theoretical Sensitivity*. Mill Valley, California: Sociology Press.

Glaser, B. (1992) *Basics of Grounded Theory Analysis*. Mill Valley, CA: Sociology Press.

Glaser, B. and A. Strauss (1967) *The Discovery of Grounded Theory: Strategies for Qualitative Research*. Chicago: Aldine.

Harding, S. (1989) Feminist justificatory strategies, in: A. Garry and M. Pearsall (eds), *Women Knowledge and Reality: Explorations in Feminist Philosophy*. Mass.: Unwin Hyman: 189–201.

Hartsock, N. (1983) *Money, Sex and Power: Towards a Feminist Historical Materialism*. New York: Longman.

Hartsock, N. (1987) The feminist standpoint: developing the ground for a specifically feminist historical materialism, in: S. Harding (ed.), *Feminism and Methodology: Social Science Issues*. Milton Keynes: Open University Press.

Hyde, A. (1996) 'Unmarried Women's Experiences of Pregnancy and the Early Weeks of Motherhood in an Irish Context: A Qualitative Analysis', Unpublished PhD thesis, Trinity College, University of Dublin.

Illich, I. (1976) *Limits to Medicine: Medical Nemesis, the Expropriation of Health*. Harmondsworth: Penguin.

Kiely, G. (1995) Fathers in families, in I.C. McCarthy (ed.), *Irish Family Studies: Selected Papers*. Dublin: Family Studies Centre, University College, Dublin: 147–58.

Lupton, D. (1994) *Medicine as Culture: Illness, Disease and the Body in Western Societies*. London: Sage.

Macintyre, S. (1977) *Single and Pregnant*. London: Croom Helm.

Macintyre, S. (1991) Who wants babies? The social construction of instincts, in: D. Leonard and S. Allen (eds), *Sexual Divisions Revisited*. London: Macmillan: 1–24.

Market Research Bureau of Ireland (1992) *Mna na hEireann*. Dublin: MRBI.

McKee, L. (1982) Fathers' participation in infant care: a critique, in: L. McKee and M. O'Brien (eds), *The Father Figure*. London: Tavistock: 120–38.

Murphy-Lawless, J. (1988a) The silencing of women in childbirth or let's hear it for Bartholomew and the boys, *Women's Studies International Forum*, 11 (4): 293–8.

Murphy-Lawless, J. (1988b) 'Women and Childbirth: Male Medical Discourse and the Invention of Female Incompetence', Unpublished PhD thesis, Trinity College, University of Dublin.

Murphy-Lawless, J. (1988c) The obstetric view of feminine identity: a nineteenth century case history of the use of forceps on unmarried women in Ireland, in: A. Todd and S. Fisher (eds), *Gender and Discourse: The Power of Talk*. New Jersey: Ablex: 177–98.

Oakley, A. (1980) *Women Confined: Towards a Sociology of Childbirth*. Oxford: Martin Robertson.

O'Connor, P. (1995) Understanding continuities and changes in Irish marriage: putting women centre stage, *Irish Journal of Sociology*, 5: 135–63.

Richardson, D. (1993) *Women, Mothering and Childrearing*. London: Macmillan.

Rose, H. (1983) Hand, brain and heart: a feminist epistemology for the natural sciences, *Signs,* 9: 73–90.

Rose, H. (1986) Beyond masculinist realities: a feminist epistemology for the sciences, in R. Bleier (ed.), *Feminist Approaches to Science.* New York: Pergamon: 57–76.

Skrabanek, P. (1994) *The Death of Humane Medicine and the Rise of Coercive Healthism.* Suffolk: Social Affairs Unit.

Smith, D.E. (1979) A sociology for women, in: J. Sherman and E. Beck (eds), *The Prism of Sex: Essays in the Sociology of Knowledge.* Madison: University of Wisconsin Press: 135–87.

Smith, D.E. (1987) *The Everyday World as Problematic: A Feminist Sociology.* Milton Keynes: Open University Press.

Strauss, A.L. (1987) *Qualitative Analysis for Social Scientists.* Cambridge: Cambridge University Press.

Strauss, A.L. and J. Corbin (1990) *Basics of Qualitative Research: Grounded Theory Procedures and Techniques.* London: Sage.

Strauss, A.L. and J. Corbin (1994) Grounded theory methodology: an overview, in N. Denzin and Y. Lincoln (eds), *Handbook of Qualitative Research.* London: Sage.

Zola, I.K. (1972) Medicine as an institution of social control, *Sociological Review,* 20: 487–504.

8

Beyond the Moral Panic – Results from a Recent Study of Teenage Pregnancy

Andrew Finlay, Dorothy Whittington, Nicola Shaw, and Monica McWilliams

Introduction

This chapter reports on research which was carried out between March 1992 and December 1993. The research was commissioned by the Western Health and Social Services Board (WHSSB) in Northern Ireland (NI). Although the study was confined to the WHSSB area,[1] the chapter concludes by locating the findings in relation to trends in the rest of NI, in the Republic of Ireland and in Britain.

Let us begin with the context in which the research was commissioned and carried out. A subdued moral panic about teenage pregnancy simmered in Britain through much of the 1980s (Phoenix 1991: 220). The issue came to the boil following a visit to Britain in 1989 by Charles Murray, the North American social policy expert, who argues that young unmarried mothers are the dynamo for a burgeoning underclass which is undermining both family and community, is a major cause of lawlessness and a drain on the public purse (Murray, 1990). In NI teenage pregnancy became an issue in the early 1990s following the decision by the Director for Public Health at Eastern Health and Social Services Boards (EHSSB) to invite the Brook Advisory Service to set up a clinic. Brook is a British-based organisation which provides a confidential and non-judgmental advice and contraceptive service to young people. A campaign against Brook was mounted by a coalition which crossed NI's usual religious and political divisions. Most of the protagonists in the ensuing controversy – including those in favour of Brook and those against – agreed that the increasing numbers of births being registered by unmarried teenagers in NI was problematic (see Finlay and Shaw 1993).

In the context of this moral panic, public health professionals in Britain and NI have, for the most part, been careful to avoid moralistic or emotive language and to phrase their concern in technical or scientific terms (Finlay and Shaw, 1993). They tend to stress that their concern is not the fact that most pregnant teenagers are unmarried but is based on the assumption that most pregnancies to unmarried teenagers are unplanned, that most unplanned pregnancies are also unwanted and unsupported, and evidence which links such pregnancies with a range of adverse social and health outcomes for both mother and child (the evidence is discussed in a variety of publications, including: EHSSB, 1990: 30; WHSSB, 1990; Peckham, 1992; Macintyre and Cunningham-Burley, 1993).

Although medical concern tends to revolve around the supposedly unplanned, unwanted and unsupported nature of teenage pregnancy, this is not the only concern articulated by health professionals. In the course of the Brook controversy, a dissident Medico-Legal Enquiry Group emerged which claimed that the real problem was not teenage pregnancy as such but adolescent sexual activity. Moreover, the influential Health of the Nation White Paper (1992) focused particular concern on pregnancies to girls under the age of 16.

Public discourse on teenage pregnancy in the Republic of Ireland reveals some differences to that in Britain and NI. Arguably, the issue has not been as fraught in the Republic of Ireland. However, in so far as the issue has been discussed, some interesting variations in terminology are revealed.[2] For example, the phrase 'unplanned pregnancy' is not much used in the Republic of Ireland where the preferred term is 'crisis pregnancy'. This difference in terminology possibly reflects the differential impact of the family planning movement in the United Kingdom and in the Republic of Ireland.[3] Despite these differences, many of the concerns articulated in the UK have found an echo in the Republic of Ireland.

Research Aims and Strategy

In the light of the concerns expressed by health professionals, a main aim of our research was to explore the extent to which pregnancies to unmarried teenagers were, in fact, unplanned, unwanted and unsupported. In addition to this we sought to gather information on the reproductive behaviour and knowledge of teenagers in relation to their social and cultural milieu, the social networks of support available to teenagers during and immediately after their pregnancies and on teenagers' use of relevant health and social services.

We also hoped that the data collected on patterns of reproductive behaviour (sexual activity, contraceptive use, family formation and so forth) would inform discussion of broader issues. Although the study was not aimed at explaining why the number of births to unmarried teenagers had increased in the past ten years it was hoped that the findings would illuminate this broader question.

The study had several elements: a virtual census of women under the age of 20 attending ante-natal clinics in the study-area between 1 September 1992 and 1 September 1993 (N=276), semi-structured interviews with sub-samples of these women during their pregnancy (N=62) and after their pregnancy had reached its outcome (N=32), and semi-structured interviews with the fathers of children born to some of the latter (N=8).

There are advantages and disadvantages to this strategy. The main advantage is that we were able to ensure that the sub-samples of women with whom we conducted semi-structured. interviews were broadly representative of all pregnant teenagers reporting to ante-natal clinics in the study area. The brief questionnaire used in the census sought to elicit information about the main socio-demographic characteristics of women under the age of 20 attending ante-natal clinics in the study-area. It was administered by midwives. The women with whom we conducted semi-structured interviews were selected on a quota basis using the information gathered by the midwives. Our quota sample was constructed using the following criteria: age, marital status, social class, religion, area of residence. It should be noted that participation in the study was voluntary and by informed consent, and that refusals to participate in the study were monitored for potential bias.

The main disadvantage of this strategy is that it effectively excluded pregnant teenagers who opt for abortion. It would seem that women who are seriously thinking about terminating their pregnancy do not usually present at ante-natal clinics; certainly, out of the 62 women with whom we conducted semi-structured interviews, only one opted for abortion.

As will become apparent, the fact that we did not sample all pregnant teenagers but, for the most part, only those who intended to go to term and the fact that we know little about women who opt for abortion are limiting factors in the interpretation of some of our findings. One further caveat: a sample like ours is not a sound basis from which to make generalisations about adolescent sexual activity more generally, as our respondents were, by definition, sexually active.

Findings

Socio-Demographic Characteristics of Teenagers Presenting at Ante-Natal Clinics

Only four (1.4%) of the teenagers were under the age of 16; most (66%) were aged 18 or 19. However, it is noteworthy that 14% of respondents were under the age of 17, the legal age of consent in NI. Most teenagers (82%) described themselves as being in an ongoing relationship, but only 28% were married or engaged; even fewer (15%) were cohabiting. The putative fathers tended to be slightly older than their female partners: 60% were between the ages of 20 and 24, 31% were under the age of 20 and only 6.3% were aged 25 or over.

In Britain and the USA, early motherhood is less common among middle-class women (those of higher socio-economic status) than among working-class women (those of lower socio-economic status). This is also true for the Western Board: 58% of women presenting at ante-natal clinics described themselves as poor or working class and only 8% as middle class (the balance is made up of 'don't knows'). Most women were in employment or full-time education (36% and 19% respectively); however, 41% described themselves as unemployed or 'keeping house'.

Data from Britain and the USA also suggest that rates of teenage motherhood may vary among teenagers from different cultural groups. This also seems to be the case in the Western Board area: Catholic women are slightly over-represented, and Protestant women under-represented, relative to their numbers in the general population of women aged 14 to 19.

We would remind the reader that the above data relate to pregnant teen-agers presenting at ante-natal clinics rather than to all teenagers who conceive. The latter include an indeterminate number who opt for abortion, and, as we have seen, most of these do not present at ante-natal clinics. Available statistics relating to women from NI having abortions in Britain are not broken down by religious affiliation, social class or area of residence. Because of this, the data presented above should be interpreted with caution, particularly with regard to ethnicity and class. With regard to the latter, it is noteworthy that evidence from elsewhere suggests that middle-class women are more likely to have abortions than their working class counterparts (Dawson, 1996: 6). With regard to ethnicity, it should be stressed that the data do not necessarily mean that the conception rate is higher among teenagers from a Catholic background than among those from a Protestant background; e.g. it may be that Protestant teenagers are more likely to opt for abortion than Catholic teenagers. However, the semi-structured interviews with pregnant teenagers revealed surprisingly few differences in knowledge and attitudes to abortion and contraception among Catholic and Protestant teenagers (cf. West *et al.*, 1993)

Antecedents of Pregnancy

Of the 62 women with whom we conducted in-depth interviews, virtually all had received some kind of sex education at school, and most (more than 75%) mentioned having 'a talk' about sex with one of their parents, usually their mother. Sex education in schools, as described by our respondents, was remarkably varied in terms of the way it had been delivered and the time devoted to it, but for most respondents it was felt to be either too little or too late. It is particularly noteworthy that contraceptive information was commonly omitted from the sex education which our respondents received at school and in the home (not mentioned in 50% and 63% of cases respectively). An exception to this fairly dismal picture of sex education in schools was where professional health educators from outside the school had been involved.

Despite the perceived inadequacy of sex education in general and contraceptive education in particular, our respondents were not ignorant about how conception occurs and the main methods of preventing it; however, there was some confusion about natural methods of birth control and uncertainty about the contraceptive pill. All respondents were by definition sexually active, but few could be described as promiscuous: 70% claimed they were aged 16 or over when they first had sexual intercourse, 45% indicated that the putative father had been their first sexual partner and most pregnancies (69%) occurred within the context of an ongoing relationship of at least six months duration. Only one respondent said that she became pregnant as the result of a casual encounter and only 16% admitted to having had three or more sexual partners. Moreover, although all respondents were sexually active, in the sense that they had had sexual intercourse, this does not necessarily indicate a lot of sexual activity: for many (up to 80%) sexual intercourse was an irregular occurrence: something which 'just happened' when they had the necessary privacy.

Family Planning

Contemporary discussion of teenage pregnancy tends to be polarised between those – mainly health professionals – who assume that most pregnancies to unmarried women under the age of 20 are *unplanned*, and those, such as Charles Murray, who suggest that many young women *plan* their pregnancies in order to gain access to public housing and welfare benefits.[4] Neither of these stereotypes accurately represent our respondents. Indeed, our respondents' experiences cannot be captured in terms of a simple dichotomy between planned and unplanned pregnancy (see Finlay 1996 for a fuller critique of this dichotomy). Their accounts of how they came to be pregnant are complex and nuanced. Thus, while it is possible to classify approximately 40 (65%) of the pregnancies as unplanned and 10 (16%) as planned, the remainder defy such classification: some women described their pregnancies as 'sort of planned', others indicated that they had wanted a baby at some time in their lives and it 'didn't matter' when.

Of the 40 respondents whose pregnancies can be classified as unplanned, 15 claimed that they had been consistent in their use of some form of birth control and attributed their pregnancy to its failure. The remaining 25 respondents said that they had not been using any method of birth control consistently or ever. They usually had well-rehearsed explanations as to why they had not been using any method of birth control. The contraceptive pill often featured.

One of the most common explanations was that they had been discouraged from getting the contraceptive pill for fear of people, particularly their mothers, finding out. Another common explanation involved the contraceptive pill and its real or supposed side effects: either the respondent had stopped taking the pill because of side-effects or had been discouraged from getting the contraceptive pill because she had been told about its side-effects. Other explanations included the refusal of a GP to prescribe the pill without parental consent, and the refusal or inability of their sexual partner to use condoms.[5]

Explanations of why respondents persisted in having sex without contraception were more hesitant; nevertheless, it is possible to identify two main types. One type of explanation involved a denial of fertility: 'I didn't think that I would have got pregnant, I suppose everybody does at some stage, but no, not me' (153A). Hyde (1995: 25) has suggested that some young women seem to believe that they would not become pregnant until they wished to or were socially ready.

In the second type of explanation, sex is presented as something which 'just happens' in the heat of the moment. For example, one respondent explained why she continued having sex after she had stopped taking the pill in the following way:

'Just not thinking . . . me and my boyfriend were just minding somebody's house, and it [sex] just happened. We got carried away'. (039L)

Other examples include: 'it [sex] was just quick and you don't think about them things [contraception]' (001A), or 'it all went so quick you know: I didn't really think at the time' (129O). In this explanation it is possible to find echoes of the code of romantic love which Angela McRobbie (1978) and Sue Lees (1986 and 1992) suggest is pervasive in the culture of working-class girls. According to the code of romantic love, it is not acceptable for a young woman to desire or plan to have sex: having sex is only acceptable if you are in love and 'get carried away'. For a young woman to be on the pill or carrying condoms would be to 'risk savage criticism since such calculated, premeditated action totally contravenes the dominant code of romance' (McRobbie, 1978: 98). One sociologist, writing in the context of a review of research on HIV-related risk behaviour, comments that this code 'makes it preferable for some women to fall pregnant through unpremeditated sex than to go on the pill and be labelled as promiscuous' (Wight, 1992: 15). Some of our respondents claimed to have been 'carried away'; however, they did not claim to have been carried away by love. Indeed, love is notable by its absence from our respondents' explanations of how they came to be pregnant.[6]

Responses To Pregnancy

Few, if any, of our respondents' pregnancies can be described as unwanted. It is true that those who had not intended to become pregnant tended to be upset and fearful when they first realised that they were pregnant. These initial reactions suggest that a considerable degree of stigma still adheres to unmarried teenage pregnancy: in addition to anxieties about how they would cope with a child, respondents were afraid of how other people, particularly their parents, would react. This fear was most acute for younger respondents and those who did not have a partner in evidence. However, these initial fears and anxieties mellowed as the pregnancy progressed. For most respondents, telling their parents was a watershed. Thereafter, many respondents embraced impending motherhood with zeal, others wished it had not happened but were determined to make the best of their situation, only a few remained unhappy: unplanned and unwanted pregnancy are two different things.

Many of our respondents' parents reacted negatively when they learnt of their daughters' pregnancy, but virtually all accepted it and became the single most important source of financial and practical support both during the pregnancy and after its outcome. Most of our respondents were living in their parental home when they became pregnant, and most chose to remain there in preference to finding a place of their own or to cohabiting with their partner. None were asked to leave their home, though one or two left because of lack of space.

Although many of our respondents who were neither married nor cohabiting described themselves as 'going steady', these relationships were often unstable: we recorded a number of break-ups and re-formations. When relationships broke up they were more often terminated by the female rather than the male partner. In only one case did the male partner refuse to acknowledge paternity. In the majority of cases, he remained in daily contact with his partner and child, but the financial support he offered was often limited by his own lack of economic resources: most were from similar social backgrounds as their partners: 26% were in employment, 13% worked in youth and community schemes, 2% were in full-time education and 26% were unemployed (the balance are missing data).

Conclusions

The research reported in this chapter was commissioned against the background of a growing moral panic about the increasing numbers of births being registered by unmarried women under the age of twenty. In our report to the health board that commissioned the research we concluded that the panic was not warranted, at least not from the perspective of public health in the board area.

The reader will recall that much medical concern revolves around the supposedly unplanned, unwanted and unsupported nature of pregnancies to unmarried teenagers; evidence which links such pregnancies with a range of adverse health and social outcomes; and the fact that pregnancies to unmarried teenagers are increasing. Against this, we found that a significant proportion of our respondents' pregnancies were planned, that very few of those pregnancies classified as unplanned and which went to term can be described as unwanted and that most respondents received high levels of support from their families.

The numbers of women under the age of twenty who register births in the Western Board area – and in NI as a whole (see Table 1) – has not increased in the last two decades; what seems to have changed is that a larger proportion give birth out of wedlock. Our findings do not suggest that marriage has become unpopular among teenagers or that there has been a decisive shift towards cohabitation. Typically, our respondents were part of an ongoing, but fairly labile, relationship with the putative father. They wanted to get married at some time in their lives but felt little pressure to do so in the near future; in the meantime they preferred to live at their parental home.

Table 1 *Legitimate and illegitimate births registered by women under the age of 20 in Northern Ireland 1974–1993*

Year	Legitimate	Illegitimate	Total	Illegitmate births as a percentage of the total number of births
1974	1799	453	2252	20.1
1975	1828	464	2292	20.2
1976	2126	465	2591	17.9
1977	1573	491	2064	23.8
1978	1588	539	2127	25.3
1979	1645	555	2200	25.2
1980	1553	571	2124	26.9
1981	1280	632	1912	33.1
1982	1247	666	1913	34.8
1983	1149	798	1947	41.0
1984	1069	956	2025	47.2
1985	914	1064	1978	53.8
1986	894	1202	2096	57.3
1987	731	1278	2009	63.6
1988	658	1396	2054	68.0
1989	510	1391	1901	73.2
1990	445	1413	1858	76.0
1991	325	1464	1789	81.8
1992	329	1531	1860	82.3
1993	187	1409	1596	88.3

Source: Registrar General Northern Ireland, Annual Reports (1974–1993), Belfast: HMSO.

These findings would seem to be in line with recent research carried out in Glasgow and London (for example see Macintyre and Cunningham-Burley, 1993, and Phoenix, 1991). However, our research suggests that NI may be different from Britain in some important respects.

When one hears the phrase 'teenage pregnancy' the image conjured up is that of a distressed schoolgirl. The reader will recall that the Department of Health (UK) has expressed particular concern about conceptions to teenagers under the age of 16. They have done so because 'Britain has one of the highest teenage pregnancy rates in Western Europe with conception rates amongst the under 16 rising steadily until 1991' (NHSME Communications Unit, November 1993). Because of the lack of accurate figures for women who opt for abortion, it is not possible to calculate conception rates for the study area or for NI as a whole. However, it is notable that most pregnant teenagers in the WHSSB area were aged 18 or 19 (66.6%), that only four were under the age of 16 (1.4%) and that the number of births to teenagers under the age of 16 has not increased in the last decade. Moreover, a recent study of education and employment opportunities for schoolgirl mothers states that 'based on absolute numbers of births and school population it can be inferred that NI has the lowest rate of conception to the under 16 year old (*sic*) in the UK.' (Dawson, 1996: 5).

In terms of the numbers of pregnant teenagers, their ages and trends, NI seems to be more in line with the Republic of Ireland than Britain. For example, Magee concludes her review of existing data about teenage pregnancy in the Republic of Ireland as follows:

> Many will be surprised to discover that the numbers of births to teenagers has not risen over the last twenty years and that a very small proportion of these births are to school girls. Indeed the number of births to young women under 16 was ten less in 1992 (45) than in 1972 (55). The changing marital status of these mothers may be the real source of public concern about teen parenting. In 1972, 24% of births to women under twenty were outside marriage, by 1992 it was 89.3%. (1994: 52)

All in all, our findings tend to allay the fears expressed by health professionals regarding teenage pregnancy, but they also point to particular areas of concern and are suggestive of ways in which these can be addressed. Our report to the WHSSB identified two main areas of concern. Firstly, although our data suggest that it is not safe to assume that pregnancies to unmarried teenagers are unplanned, unwanted and unsupported, the fact is that 65% of our respondents did not intend to become pregnant. Secondly, a considerable amount of stigma still adheres to teenage pregnancy. The feelings which this engenders can cause distress and can have an adverse effect on help-seeking behaviour and relations with service providers. In the light of these concerns we made a series of recommendations for policy and practice aimed at reducing unintended pregnancies and responding to the needs of women under the age of 20 who become pregnant.

A further concern is suggested by the fact that the young women who participated in the study tended to reside in areas of social deprivation. This suggestion should not be interpreted as support for Charles Murray's ideas about an underclass. We did not set out to investigate the relationship between non-marital births, unemployment, welfare, housing and crime; indeed the controversy generated by his ideas emerged after our research had been commissioned. However, in so far as the data which we collected is relevant to this controversy, it tends to contradict Murray: most of our respondents did not consciously plan their pregnancy, most were still in a relationship with the putative father, most preferred to remain in their parental home rather than seek public housing. It is true that some of the minority of respondents who had considered cohabiting with the putative father had been discouraged by the fact that he was unemployed and that if they formally lived together they would lose out on benefit. The relationship between non-marital births, unemployment, welfare and housing is more complicated than Murray allows and is worthy of further research (see Piachaud, 1997 and Wilson, 1996).

Notes

We acknowledge the assistance and support of many colleagues in the WHSSB, particularly Dr William McConnell, Mrs Stella Burnside, Mrs Elaine Way, Dr Mary McKeever and Dr Fiona Kennedy. We are also much indebted to the young people who agreed to talk to us. The views expressed in this chapter are the responsibility of the first author.

1   The WHSSB area is adjacent to the border with the Irish Republic. It is largely rural, but includes one small city, Derry or Londonderry, and several large towns.

2   The attention of those who commission social research seems to have focused more on single motherhood than on teenage pregnancy (e.g. see Flanagan and Richardson, 1992; O'Hare, c.1983; McCashin, 1996); Magee (1994) is an exception in this regard. Although teenage pregnancy has, by comparison to the UK, not attracted much research and public comment, other aspects of reproductive health have: notably contraception, abortion, and the manner in which single mothers and their babies were treated in the recent past. Further research is in progress. The first author is one of a team of researchers at Trinity College, Dublin which was recently commissioned by the Department of Health to conduct an ongoing study of women and pregnancy in Ireland (see Mahon and Conlon, 1996).

3   The notion of 'unplanned pregnancy' is a recent one. Prior to the advent of effective forms of birth control and a family planning movement which made the widespread use of these acceptable, the terms planned and unplanned pregnancy would have little meaning. In addition to the fact that reliable methods of birth control were not generally available, higher rates of infant mortality meant that babies were regarded as 'gifts from God' rather than as something one planned. In this context, to have described a pregnancy as planned would have been somewhat anomalous. Today, there is a danger that unplanned pregnancies are perceived as being anomalous. Certainly, some of the young women we interviewed felt stigmatised when the term was applied to them.

4   It is interesting that two such contradictory views of teenage pregnancy can coexist at the level of public discourse.

5   In one or two cases there were differences between what a female respondent told us and what her partner told us. These differences raise further questions about the usefulness of the terms 'planned pregnancy' and 'unplanned pregnancy'. For example, one or two of those pregnancies which we classified as unplanned on the basis of information supplied by the female respondent may not have been totally unpremeditated by their partners.

6   This absence of love from respondents' explanations, of how they came to be pregnant may be symptomatic of a 'transformation of intimacy' such as that described by Giddens (1992). Finlay (1996) explores this possibility.

References

Bury, J. (1984) *Teenage Pregnancy in Britain*. London: Birth Control Trust.

Cartwright, A. (1988) Unintended pregnancies that lead to babies, *Social Science and Medicine*, 27 (3): 249–59.

Cheetham, J. (1977) *Unwanted Pregnancy and Counselling*, London: Routledge.

Dawson, N. (1996) *The Provision of Education and Opportunities for Future Employment for Pregnant Schoolgirls and Schoolgirl Mothers*. Bristol: School of Education, University of Bristol

Department of Health (1992) *Health of the Nation*. London: Department of Health.

EHSSB Director of Public Health (1990*) Public Health Matters Annual Report 1989*, Belfast: Eastern Health and Social Service Board.

Finlay, A. and N. Shaw (1993) Brook in Belfast and the 'problem' of teenage pregnancy, *Critical Public Health*, 4, (2): 24–30.

Finlay, A., N. Shaw, D.Whittington and M. McWilliams (1995) *Adolescent Reproductive Behaviour in the Western Health and Social Services Board Area – Executive Summary*. Coleraine-Londonderry: University of Ulster/Western Health and Social Services Board: 1–8.

Finlay, A. (1996) Teenage pregnancy, romantic love and social science: an uneasy relationship, in V. James and J. Gabe (eds) *Health and the Sociology of Emotion*. Oxford: Blackwell.

Flanagan, N. and V. Richardson (1992) *Unmarried Mothers: A Social Profile*. Dublin: University College, Dublin, Department of Social Policy and Social Work/Social Science Research Centre and National Maternity Hospital, Social Work Research Unit.

Giddens, A. (1992) *The Transformation of Intimacy: Sexuality, Love and Eroticism in Modern Societies*. Cambridge: Polity.

Hudson, F. and B. Ineichen (1991) *Taking it Lying Down: Sexuality and Teenage Motherhood*. London: Macmillan.

Hyde, A. (1995) Younger and older women's contraceptive practices in the lead up to their pregnancies, *Northern Exposure, Spring Symposium of the Scottish Society of Family Planning Nurses*, Inverness.

Lees, S. (1986) *Losing Out Sexuality and Adolescent Girls*. London: Hutchinson.

Lees, S. (1992) *Sugar and Spice Sexuality and Adolescent Girls*. London: Penguin.

Magee, C (1994) *Teenage Parents Issues of Policy and Practice*. Dublin: Irish YouthWork Press.

Mahon, E. and C. Conlon (1996) Legal abortions carried out in England on women normally resident in the Republic of Ireland, Appendix 21, *Report of the Constitution Review Group*, Dublin: Stationery Office.

Macintyre, S and S. Cunningham-Burley (1993) Teenage pregnancy as a social problem: a perspective from the United Kingdom, in: A. Lawson and D.L. Rhode (eds) *The Politics of Pregnancy: Adolescent Sexuality and Public Policy*. London: Yale University Press.

McCashin, A. (1996) *Lone Mothers in Ireland: A Local Study*. Dublin: Combat Poverty Agency.

McRobbie, A. (1978) Working class girls and the culture of femininity, in: Women's Studies Group, Centre for Contemporary Cultural Studies, University of Birmingham, *Women Take Issue Aspects of Women's Subordination*. London: Hutchinson.

McRobbie, A. (1989) Motherhood a teenage job, *The Guardian*, 5 September.

McRobbie, A. (1991) *Feminism and Youth Culture From 'Jackie' to 'Just Seventeen'*. London: Macmillan.

Murray, C. (1990) *The Emerging British Under-Class*. London: IEA Health and Welfare Unit.

NHS Management Executive Communications Unit (1993) *The Health of the Nation*. Leeds.

O'Hare, A. *et al.* (*c.* 1983) *Mothers Alone: A Study of Women Who Gave Birth Outside Marriage in Ireland*. Dublin: Federation of Services for Unmarried Parents and their Children.

Peckham, S. (1992) *Unplanned Pregnancy and Teenage Pregnancy A Review.* Wessex Research Consortium, Institute for Health Policy Studies, University of Southampton.

Phoenix, A. (1991) *Young Mothers?* Cambridge: Polity Press.

Phoenix, A. (1993) The social construction of teenage motherhood: a black and white issue, in: A. Lawson and D.L. Rhode (eds) *The Politics of Pregnancy: Adolescent Sexuality and Public Policy.* London: Yale University Press.

Piachaud, D (1997) Down but not out: Why the term 'underclass' is no help in understanding social ills, *Times Literary Supplement*, 24 January: 3–4.

Registrar General Northern Ireland, *Annual Reports* (1974–1993), Belfast: HMSO.

West, P., D. Wight and S. Macintyre (1993) Heterosexual Behaviour of 18-year-olds in the Glasgow area, *Journal of Adolescence*, 16 (4): 367–96.

WHSSB Director of Public Health (1990) *Health Accounts 1989 – A Time for Change Annual Report*, Londonderry: Western Health and Social Services Board.

Wight, D. (1992) Impediments to safer heterosexual sex: a review of research with young people, *AIDS Care*, 4 (1): 11–23.

Wilson, W. J. (1996) *When Work Disappears: The World of the New Urban Poor.* New York: Knopf.

9

Contesting Concepts of Care:
The Case of the Home Help Service in Ireland

Orla O'Donovan

Introduction

Since the publication in 1983 of Finch's and Groves's influential edited
collection of essays, *A Labour of Love: Women, Work and Caring*, a considerable
amount of sociological, social policy and feminist scholarship has been devoted
to the analysis of caring. Much of the Irish research on caring over the past
decade has involved empirical studies focused on unveiling the 'costs' of caring,
including the health costs borne by carers (for example O'Connor and Ruddle,
1988; Ruddle and O'Connor, 1993; Blackwell *et al.*, 1992). A current focus of
work in this field amongst feminist researchers concerns the conceptualisation
of care. In the British feminist tradition of research on caring, there has been a
tendency to conceptualise it in terms of unpaid work performed by women for
their relatives in the home. However, in recent years, two of the 'mothers' of
that tradition, Graham (1991) and Ungerson (1990, 1995), have developed
critiques of conventional feminist conceptualisations of care and have
highlighted that the restricted boundaries of the concept have resulted in many
forms of care being excluded from feminist enquiry. Prompted by the work of
these two authors, Thomas (1993) has developed an analytical framework for
deconstructing concepts of care and has introduced a 'unified' concept that, she
claims, embraces all forms of care.

Drawing on these feminist debates about the concept of care, this chapter
explores the construction of care in health policy concerning the home help
service in Ireland. Particular reference is made to the conceptualisation of care
in the context of an ongoing debate about the training of home helps in
Ireland.[1] The chapter starts by briefly reviewing critiques of the concepts of

care that have been adopted in much feminist research on caring since the 1980s and then examines some reworked conceptualisations. An overview of the Irish home help service and the continuing debate about the training of home helps is then presented. Using the analytical framework developed by Thomas (1993), the concept of care that has been employed by the statutory health authorities in the debate about training home helps is then explored. This deconstruction of the concept of care used by the health boards highlights that their concept of care is contested by the concepts used by older people and family carers. It also serves ·to expose the health boards' policy agenda in relation to domiciliary care services for older people and the gender ideology that informs that agenda.

Reconstructing the Concept of Care

In the introduction to their seminal text on caring, Finch and Groves (1983:1) mapped out the territory of their concerns, stating that the book 'focuses upon those hundreds of thousands of women who provide unpaid care outside of residential institutions – often in their own homes – for children and adults who are handicapped or chronically sick, and for frail elderly people. Those for whom such women provide care are usually (though not invariably) relatives. . .'. Caring, therefore, was defined in terms of unpaid work performed by women for members of their family in the home. Graham examined the concept of caring in her essay in the same text and based her analysis on the distinction between the *love* and *labour* dimensions of caring, where the former dimension relates to the emotional aspects of caring and the latter relates to the service aspect. This distinction was also fundamental to Ungerson's contribution to the book, where she drew the distinction between caring *for* someone and caring *about* someone. The conceptual framework for understanding caring that was developed in this text has since been widely used in research in this field. For example, Blackwell *et al.*'s (1992: 18) study, that compared the costs of institutional and community care of older people in Ireland, acknowledged this conceptual inheritance and noted that the 'very presence of these qualities of affection and sensitivity, as Graham points out, differentiates "caring" from substitute services, and therefore makes carers and dependants unwilling to use substitute care'.

While Graham played a key role in conceptualising care as unpaid home-based kin-care provided by women, she has been to the forefront in recent calls for a reworking of the concept. Her critique of the conceptualisation of care in much feminist research is based on three related points. Firstly, she argues that feminist researchers have adopted key aspects of the concept of care used by statutory agencies in relation to community care policies. One such aspect is the merging of the location with the social relations of care by defining it as care that takes place in the home for relatives. This conceptualisation, she argues, has resulted in the obscuring of home-based care that is provided by non-relatives. Secondly, Graham argues that feminist research on caring has been based on a one-dimensional perspective on social divisions; it has focused on gender divisions and has neglected racial and class divisions. Thirdly, she argues that the concept of care used in feminist research has drawn, not always uncritically, on the concepts of the public and private spheres. Taking these three aspects of the conceptualisation of care together, she notes that the concept that defines care in terms of women's unpaid work in the private domain of the family may be useful in considering the experiences of many white women. However, she argues that it is less useful when considering much of the home-based care provided by many black women, as, in the case of domestic service in Britain and the USA, this has involved paid work in the homes of non-relatives. In thus highlighting the 'restricted focus' of the concept of care, she points to the need to reconstruct the concept so that other forms of care are included in the programme of feminist research.

In Ungerson's (1990, 1995) recent analyses of the concept of care, she presents a critique of the conventional usage in research on caring of the dichotomy between 'informal' and 'formal' care. Abrams (1978), in his study of neighbourhood care networks, is credited with having introduced this distinction, where informal care is defined as unpaid care based on personal relationships and formal care is defined as paid care that is provided within a framework of bureaucratic rules and regulations. Abrams suggested that not only are these two types of care different but, essentially, that informal care is superior to formal care because it has an emotional quality that is absent from informal care (Robertson Elliot, 1996). In Ungerson's 1990s revisiting of the concept of care she argues that formal and informal care are not necessarily qualitatively different and that both can contain aspects of both labour and love. Furthermore, while acknowledging calls in feminist literature for a dissolution of the conceptual boundaries between formal and informal care, Ungerson (1995) has more recently pointed to the introduction of state payments for carers as an example of how the empirical boundaries between these two forms of care are being removed. On this point regarding the dichotomisation of formal and informal care, Stacey (1988) has long argued that a considerable amount of care takes place in the 'intermediate zone' between the domestic and public domains. Indeed, as will be seen later in this chapter, the Irish home help service occupies this zone.

In her review of Graham's and Ungerson's reworkings of the concept of care, Thomas (1993) has argued that while these authors have extended the boundaries of care, their revised concepts are incomplete. As a result of scrutinising concepts of care that were used in feminist, social policy and government literature, she identified seven dimensions that are common to all concepts of care. She points out that variations in relation to these seven dimensions result in varying concepts of care. Her examination of variations in these dimensions then forms the basis of her 'unified' concept which, she claims, embraces all forms of care. Table 1 provides an outline of Thomas's seven dimensions of care and her all-embracing concept.

Table 1 *Thomas's (1993) framework for analysing concepts of care and her unified concept*

Seven dimensions of care	A unified concept
social identity of the carer	defined in terms of: gender (mainly, but not exclusively, women)
social identity of the care recipient	able-bodied and dependent adults and children
inter-personal relationship between carer and care recipient	familial, friends, neighbours and contingent lay and professional
nature of care	work activities (labour) and feeling states (love)
social domain	public or private
economic relationship	unwaged or waged
institutional setting	various e.g. home and a range of social service and health service settings

The first of the dimensions of the concept of care, identified by Thomas, is the social identity of the carer. As mentioned above, one of Graham's criticisms of the conventional concept of care in feminist research is the exclusive focus on gender as the social identifier of carers. In her unified concept, Thomas maintains that gender is the primary social identifier, but notes that caring is not exclusively provided by women. The second dimension relates to the social characteristics of the recipients of care. In this regard, Thomas notes the tendency in concepts of care to focus on the 'dependency status' of the care recipient. Able-bodied and 'dependent' adults and children are included in her unified concept. The relationship between the carer and the recipient of care constitutes the third dimension. We saw above that Graham was critical of the restricted focus on care provided by and to relatives. In her unified concept, Thomas includes kin/friends/neighbours and *contingent* caring relationships, where the latter are relationships between care recipients and carers that are formed in the context of the provision of specific health and social services. The fourth dimension is the nature of care; Thomas includes both feeling states or *love,* and work activities or *labour* in her unified concept. The social domain within which caring takes place is the fifth element of concepts of care identified by Thomas, and this relates to the social division of labour into the public and private spheres. Thomas includes both spheres in her concept and notes that the tendency in research on caring has been to focus on informal care or care in the private domain. The sixth dimension relates to the economic aspect of care and Thomas includes both waged and unwaged care in her concept. The final dimension relates to the setting in which care is delivered. Thomas's unified concept includes the home, in addition to a range of health and social service settings. Thomas argues that variations in these dimensions of the concept have to be teased out in order to understand the differences in various concepts of care. In her deconstruction of the revised concepts of care presented by Graham (1991) and Ungerson (1990), Thomas (1993: 660) argues that while both of them have extended the boundaries of the concept, they have done so in different directions. She argues that this reflects their varying academic agendas, where 'Graham is basically interested in the further development of a feminist theoretical understanding of the reproduction of the family, while Ungerson is concerned with care policy and the possibilities for feminist forms of care which ensure the provision of quality care for recipients without the exploitation of women'.

My purpose here is to use Thomas's framework to explore the concept of care used by the health boards in relation to the home help service, and in turn to show how this conceptualisation is linked to their policy agenda in relation to services for older people and is informed by a patriarchal gender ideology. Before doing this, however, the next section provides an overview of the home help service and reviews the debate about the training of home helps.

The Home Help Service and the Debate About Training

The home help service was established as a statutory service under Section 61 of the Health Act 1970. Under the Act, health boards are empowered (not obliged) to provide a discretionary home help service for sick or infirm people or their dependants, women who have recently given birth or their dependants and people who would otherwise need institutional care. In practice, older people constitute the largest category of clients of the service; in 1993, 83% of clients were older people. While there are no formal criteria for eligibility, indeed criteria vary from one region to the next, the existence of support from family or neighbours frequently disqualifies people from eligibility (Lundström and McKeown, 1994). In a circular issued by the Department of Health shortly after the establishment of the service, the model home help was described as follows: 'the typical recruit would be a middle-aged woman with time to spare from her other household duties who was attracted to the idea of helping to normalise the living conditions of a person or family in need of care' (Department of Health, 1972). This model of the ideal home help was recently endorsed by health boards, where they indicated that home helps 'should ideally be caring and capable mature women who have some experience of caring and whose interest in the work is not determined primarily by the level of pay' (Lundström and McKeown, 1994: 156).

When the home help service was established, the role of the home help was envisaged as being concerned with 'normal household duties (e.g. laying fires, making a light meal, cleaning the house, making beds, getting messages)' (Department of Health, 1972). Lundström and McKeown, however, found that the range of tasks performed in 1993 was much broader than the domestic tasks originally envisaged and that in four of the eight health board regions in the country, home helps provided personal care (e.g. assisting in the management of incontinence, lifting and giving prescribed medicine). This involvement of home helps in the provision of personal care is a contentious issue with health boards because it raises questions about the occupational division of labour between social care staff (such as home helps and nursing aides) and qualified nurses. Health boards have adopted varying policies regarding personal care; in some regions, a new category of personnel, the home care attendant, has been introduced specifically to perform personal care tasks. These home care attendants receive training and are better paid than home helps.

The National Council for the Elderly's recent study of the home help service in Ireland highlighted that the service has expanded considerably since its establishment, with the numbers of home helps increasing from 5,206 to 10,599 between 1978 and 1993 (Lundström and McKeown, 1994). The study also highlighted that employment in the home help service can be characterised as a secondary labour market; less than one per cent were employed on a full-time basis and the rates of pay to part-time home helps ranged from £1.00 per hour in the Western Health Board to £3.50 in the Midland Health Board. Furthermore, of the 10,599 home helps employed in the home help service in 1993, only 68 were men.

The National Council for the Elderly's study brought to the fore a long standing debate concerning the training of home helps. The study found that the service in Ireland is considerably more cost-effective than similar services in Britain and Sweden, but that this 'is achieved by less expenditure on staff salaries, inferior conditions of employment and a lack of investment in training' (Lundström and McKeown, 1994). Arising from the finding that there is minimal provision of training for home helps, the views of representatives of the eight health boards in the country were sought on the merits of establishing a nationally recognised qualification for home helps. Three of the health boards indicated that they would be supportive of such an initiative, but the remaining five of the health boards reported that they would not support such a training initiative. Opposition to the training of home helps was based on the three arguments that training was unnecessary as home helps already possess the skills required to perform their duties, that training would result in professionalisation that would threaten the voluntary or 'good neighbourly' ethos of the service and that it would cause an escalation of costs, brought about by claims for increased wages.

The debate about the training of home helps emerged as one of the key themes at the conference at which the findings of the study on the home help service were presented. In his review of the issues that arose from the study, Kieran McKeown (one of the researchers who conducted the study) argued that the debate about training raised the question 'of whether the home help service is – or at least should aspire to be – a professional service or simply a good neighbour service. What model informs the home help service: "volunteerism" or "professionalism"?' (National Council for the Elderly 1995: 15). The voluntarist model of the home help service was advocated by one of the health board representatives who addressed the conference. He outlined the special voluntary ethos of the service and suggested that home helps have charitable motives for their involvement in the service as they 'see their role as providing a personal service by helping people less fortunate than themselves' and that they benefit personally 'from providing the service, from being needed, and by sharing with others in the community' (National Council for the Elderly 1995: 20). Another speaker at the conference, who represented the National Association of Home Care Organisers, argued that training would be beneficial on a number of fronts, including improving home helps' commitment to their work, improving the quality of care and reducing the high turnover of staff in the service.

Despite the reservations of some health boards, training for home helps emerged as one of the National Council for the Elderly's central recommendations from the study of the home help service. A recommendation for the provision of education and training for social care workers in general who work with older people, subsequently formed an element of the National Council for the Elderly's submission to the Irish government's National Economic and Social Forum (National Council for the Elderly, 1994). Here, it was argued that a substantial input into education and training for carers is a requirement for the expansion and development of community support services for older people.

In order to advance the debate about the training of home helps, the National Council for the Elderly commissioned the Centre for Health Promotion Studies in University College Galway to conduct a study that would involve eliciting the views of various interest groups on a proposed national training initiative for carers of older people (O'Donovan *et al.* 1997). As part of this study, interviews were conducted with older people and family carers who had contact of some form with social care services. A key finding from these interviews was that older people and family carers tended to frame the training debate primarily in terms of the quality of care; the concerns of the health boards that had dominated the debate were not amongst the primary concerns of these two groups. Training provision for family carers and paid carers, such as home helps and nursing aides, was addressed in these interviews, but given that the focus of this discussion is on home helps, I refer here only to the findings in relation to paid carers.

The vast majority (88%) of the older people who were interviewed reported that they thought that carers, such as home helps, who work with older people, should have some kind of training. A smaller proportion, but still the majority of the older people (60%), reported that they felt this training should be mandatory. The reason most frequently given by the older people for being in favour of training carers was that it would contribute to improving the quality of care. Specific ways in which they felt it would improve the quality of care included improving the motivation of carers and their sensitivity to older people. A further related reason that was given was that training would instil more confidence in carers on the part of older people. Ways in which family carers would benefit from the training of carers, such as home helps, that were identified by the older people, included that it would improve their capacity to provide advice and to act as respite workers. Of the 40% of older people who were either uncertain or opposed to mandatory training for paid carers, the main reason given was that it might restrict the involvement in social care of some existing workers who are very competent carers. Another reason for opposing mandatory training that was mentioned by the older people was that because of the poor pay levels it would be unreasonable to expect carers to obtain training.

Eighty-six per cent of the family carers who were interviewed were in favour of some kind of training for carers and 52% reported that they felt that this training should be mandatory. As among the older people, the main reason given by the family carers for being in favour of training was that it would improve the quality of care. Many of the family carers emphasised the need to provide carers, such as home helps, with training in personal care skills in order to improve the quality of care for older people, but also to facilitate their greater involvement in personal care provision. The following extract from an interview with one of the family carers typifies this position:

> Without training people don't know how to handle old people properly . . . they hurt them if they're moving them up and down the bed . . . some people are very rough . . . training would stop this. By right, you need training for that sort of thing.
> . . .
>
> My mother is embarrassed when I do her personal care . . . it would be much better if there was someone from outside who could do it . . . it would be better for her and for me.
> (O'Donovan *et al.* 1997: 72–3)

Again as among the older people, the main concern that the family carers expressed in relation to the introduction of mandatory training for carers was that it may have negative implications for untrained people currently working in the field.

In summary, therefore, the interviews with the older people and family carers found that there was a very high level of support for the provision of training for carers, such as home helps, and that there was substantial support for this training to be made mandatory. The primary reason given by both groups for being in favour of the training was that it would contribute to improving the quality of care. Concerns about the introduction of mandatory training centred around the possible negative implications of such an initiative for existing untrained personnel.

Deconstructing the Health Boards' Concept of Care

Prior to deconstructing the health boards' concept of care that underpins the home help service, it is necessary to note that in the absence of detailed legislation in relation to the service, the operation of the home help service varies from one health board region to the next. Indeed, it was noted above that while Lundström and McKeown found that the majority of health boards were opposed to training home helps, three were in favour. Despite the fact that many aspects of the home help service are shared by the health boards, it could, therefore, be argued that the concept of care used in relation to the home help service can vary from region to region. These variations in particular dimensions of the concept are addressed below.

Table 2 *The health boards' concept of care*

Seven dimensions of care	
social identity of the carer	economically dependent women
social identity of the care recipient	frail older people without family support
interpersonal relationship between carer and care recipient	non-familial but 'good neighbourly'
nature of care	non-work
	labour (domestic work/personal care) and *love*
social domain	private
economic relationship	paid-volunteering
institutional setting	home

Table 2 outlines the concept of care used by the health boards in relation to the seven dimensions identified by Thomas (1993). Gender is key to the social identity of home helps, as specified by the health boards and the Department of Health. This is reflected in the recruitment patterns to the service, as in

1993, less than one per cent of home helps in Ireland were men. As discussed above, the ideal home help was described in a Department of Health circular as being a mature housewife with time on her hands. Here it can be seen that the care provided by home helps is constructed by the health boards as an extension of the care they provide to their own families as wives and mothers. The gender identity of home helps is central to the debate about training, as the argument made by the health boards that home helps do not need training because they are already competent can be seen to be based on the assumption that the skills required to care for older people come naturally to women, or are an inherent aspect of femininity. The assumption that caring comes naturally to women is challenged by the findings from the interviews with the older people and family carers, as exemplified in the case of immobile older people being physically hurt when being moved by untrained carers. It has been widely noted in feminist literature that caring is constructed as the expression of femininity; indeed, O'Connor (1992) has claimed that this is particularly the case in Ireland, where the vast majority of married women are not in paid employment. In 1994, the principal economic status of 65% of married women was involvement in 'home duties', compared with 32% who were in the paid labour force (Labour Force Survey, 1995). In this regard, Mahon (1994) has argued that, until recently, Ireland could be characterised as a private patriarchy and has highlighted how the state has actively discouraged women from participating in the paid labour force.

A further and related desirable social characteristic of home helps that was highlighted by many of the health boards in the course of the Lundström and McKeown study and the training debate was that they should be philanthropic; their primary motivation for being involved in the service should be to help 'people less fortunate than themselves' rather than monetary reward. Indeed, those opposed to the training of home helps argued that training would undermine this philanthropy or 'good neighbourliness'. Gender, therefore, is not the only social identifier of the carer in the health boards' concept of care in relation to the home help service. Economic status is a related identifier, as home helps are not expected to be 'breadwinners' but, rather, are expected to be economically dependent. This conflation of gender and economic identities and the resultant perpetuation of women's economic dependency by social policies has been identified as a key feature of the patriarchal welfare state (Pateman, 1992).

In the health boards' concept of care, the two key aspects of the social identity of the recipient of care from the home help service are dependency status and level of 'informal' support. Older people constitute the vast majority of the users of the home help service and, while not uniformly so, Lundström and McKeown found that the presence of family support can disqualify people from eligibility. This can be interpreted as being based on the assumption that care provided by family is superior and/or that it does not need to be supported.

This is another dimension where the health boards' concept of care is at odds with those of the older people and family carers who were interviewed. Given that a key argument that was made by the older people and family carers in favour of the training of home helps focused on how training would improve the potential for home helps to act as respite workers, it is clear that they did not share the health boards' view of the social identity of the care recipient as older people without family support.

The inter-personal relationship between the home help and the user of the home help service that is assumed in the health boards' concept of care is non-familial but 'good neighbourly'. As was seen in the discussion above, one of the key objections to training home helps made by health boards related to concern with the potential impact of training on this 'neighbourly' relationship. This argument is rooted in the assumptions that a voluntarist type service has a strong emotional dimension and that training would diminish the quality of the caring relationship by reducing the 'caring about' or 'love' element. The older people and family carers were less likely to construct the relationship between the home help and the care recipient as 'good neighbourly'. Indeed, their arguments that training would improve the motivation and sensitivity of home helps prompts one to question how *good* this 'good neighbourly' service actually is. This assumption that there is a strong love element in the 'good neighbourly' home help service is also called into question by the contribution from the National Association of Home Care Organisers to the training debate where it was argued that training would contribute to improving the commitment of home helps to their work and reducing the high turnover of staff.

Clearly, the repeated evocation of the 'good neighbourly' aspect of the service can be interpreted as an understanding that the nature of care involves *love*. With regard to the *labour* aspect, it is necessary to address the distinction that is drawn between domestic work and personal care, where the latter involves types of care that fall into the blurred boundaries in the occupational division of labour between nursing and social care. When the home help service was established, it was envisaged that the nature of the care that would be provided would be assistance with domestic tasks only. However, as Lundström and McKeown found, in many health board areas home helps also provide personal care. The argument made by the older people and the family carers that training would facilitate the extension of the service to include more personal care, suggests that they see the labour aspect as embracing both domestic work and personal care. Furthermore, when considering the nature of the care provided by home helps, it is clear that the health boards construct it as non-work. This conferring of the status of non-work to care provided by the home help service is evident in the comments made by the health board official who advocated the voluntarist model at the conference that discussed the findings of the study of the home help service described above. He suggested that the home help service is a charitable activity from which home helps benefit by 'being needed'. This construction of the care provided by home helps as non-work is also reflected in the rates of pay for home helps. In her discussion of housework, Oakley (1974) addressed this social trivialisation of women's work (and women) and related it to the social construction of femininity where home and family are primary, unlike the construction of masculine identity where work is primary.

The very name of the home help service indicates the social domain in which the health boards envisage this type of care taking place, namely, the private domain of the home. This relates, however, to the social domain of the care recipient, as 'home' in this instance is the work place, or public domain, of the home help. The economic basis of the relationship between home helps and the users of the service does not fall neatly into either the waged or unwaged categories in Thomas's model. As noted above, payments to home helps were as low as £1 per hour in one health board region in 1993. These rates of pay suggest that the home help service is perceived by the health boards as a form of paid volunteering and that the payments are what Ungerson (1995: 39) calls 'quasi-wages', where 'these payments are symbolic and unrelated to market levels of wages, but, like wages, are conditional on certain tasks being fulfilled and subject to formal and informal contract'. Finally, the institutional setting in which care is provided by the home help service is, clearly, confined to the home.

Conclusion

Population projections for Ireland for the period 1991 to 2011 predict that that there will be relatively slow population ageing, but that there will be dramatic changes in the composition of the older population (Fahey, 1995). It is predicted that there will be an increase of two-thirds in the numbers of people aged 80 years and over; these are the older people who are most likely to be in need of care. Similar to other European countries, health policy in relation to older people in Ireland has been dominated by the rhetoric of community care for at least a decade. The most recent health strategy, *Shaping a Healthier Future – A Strategy for Effective Health Care in the 1990s* (Department of Health, 1992) included a target that by 1997, not less than 90% of people aged 75 years and over continue to live at home. Despite this rhetoric, community-based services for older people remain largely low-status and under-resourced. The home help service provides an example of the lack of commitment to resourcing community-based services to older people in Ireland. Despite repeated calls from agencies such as the National Council for the Elderly to establish it as a core service underpinned by legislation and appropriate statutory funding, it remains a discretionary service. In 1993, only 3.5% of older people in Ireland were in receipt of the home help service (National Council for the Elderly, 1995).

As can be seen from the discussion in this chapter, this policy agenda of promoting care of older people in the 'community', but not resourcing this care, is clearly reflected in the concept of care that is used by statutory health authorities. The analysis of the concept of care that is used in relation to the home help service also exposes the gender ideology that informs this policy agenda. As we have seen, 'care' has been constructed in this instance as charitable non-work provided by philanthropic women to their less fortunate neighbours. Returning to the concern expressed by Graham (1991) about the restricted focus of research on care, this discussion highlights the importance of not only studying unpaid home-based kin-care when attempting to develop knowledge of the oppression of women by the patriarchal welfare state. Consideration also needs to be given to employees and quasi-employees, as in the case of home helps, of the welfare state who provide care. Furthermore, consideration needs to be given to the recipients of care, as, in the case of services for older people, most of these are also women.

Notes

[1]   This debate about training carers is by no means confined to Ireland. Jamieson (1991), in her review of domiciliary care services for older people in Europe, reports that they are predominantly provided by untrained women and that there are very few national standards or requirements for training. She notes that this lack of training is increasingly being viewed as problematic, particularly in the light of the trend across Europe of a shift in the division of labour between qualified nurses and carers, such as home helps, where the latter are not only involved in domestic work but also have responsibilities in relation to personal care service provision.

References

Abrams, P. (1978) *Neighbourhood Care and Social Policy*. Berkhamsted: Volunteer Centre.

Blackwell, J., E. O'Shea, G. Moane and P. Murray (1992) *Care Provision and Cost Measurement: Dependent Elderly People at Home and in Geriatric Hospitals*. Dublin: Economic and Social Research Institute.

Department of Health (1972) *Home Help Service: Circular 11/72*. Dublin: Department of Health.

Department of Health (1992*) Shaping a Healthier Future – A Strategy for Effective Healthcare in the 1990s*. Dublin: Stationery Office.

Fahey, T. (1995*) Health and Social Care Implications of Population Ageing in Ireland 1991–2011*. Dublin: National Council for the Elderly.

Finch, J. and D. Groves (eds) (1983) *A Labour of Love: Women, Work and Caring*. London: Routledge.

Graham, H. (1983) Caring: a labour of love, in: J. Finch and D. Groves, *A Labour of Love: Women, Work and Caring*, London: Routledge.

Graham, H. (1991) The concept of caring in feminist research: the case of domestic service, *Sociology*, 25 (1): 61–78.

Jamieson, A. (1991) *Home Care for Older People in Europe*. Oxford: Oxford University Press.

Labour Force Survey (1995) *Labour Force Survey*. Dublin: Stationery Office.

Lundström, F. and K. McKeown (1994) *Home Help Services for Elderly People in Ireland*. Dublin: National Council for the Elderly.

Mahon, E. (1994) Ireland – A Private Patriarchy?, *Environment and Planning*, 26: 1277–96.

National Council for the Elderly (1994) *Older People in Ireland: Social Problem or Human Resource? A Submission to the National Economic and Social Forum*. Dublin: National Council for the Elderly.

National Council for the Elderly (1995) *Home Help Services for Elderly People in Ireland: Proceedings of Conference*. Dublin: National Council for the Elderly.

Oakley, A. (1974) *Housewife*. London: Allen and Unwin.

O'Connor, J. and H. Ruddle (1988) *Caring for the Elderly, Part II – The Caring Process: A Study of Carers in the Home*. Dublin: National Council for the Aged.

O'Connor, P. (1992) The professionalisation of child care work in Ireland: an unlikely development? *Children and Society*, 6 (3): 250–66.

O'Donovan, O., M. Hodgins, V. McKenna and C. Kelleher (1997) *Training Carers of Older People: An Advisory Report*. Dublin: National Council for the Elderly.

Robertson Elliot, F. (1996) *Gender, Family and Society*. London: Macmillan.

Ruddle, H. and J. O'Connor (1993) *Caring Without Limits: Sufferers of Dementia/ Alzheimer's Disease: A Study of their Carers.* Dublin: Alzheimer's Society of Ireland.

Stacey, M. (1988) *The Sociology of Health and Healing.* London: Routledge.

Thomas, C. (1993) De-constructing concepts of care, *Sociology*, 27 (4): 649–69.

Ungerson, C. (1983) Why do women care? in: J. Finch and D. Groves (eds) *A Labour of Love: Women, Work and Caring.* London: Routledge.

Ungerson, C. (1990) *Gender and Caring: Work and Welfare in Britain and Scandinavia.* London: Harvester Wheatsheaf.

Ungerson, C. (1995) Gender, cash and informal care; European perspectives and dilemmas, *Journal of Social Policy*, 24 (1): 31–52.

10

Older People and Life-Course Construction in Ireland

Ricca Edmondson

The process of growing older has changed radically in Ireland during the last half century. At the beginning of that period, possessing a modicum of economic independence – a small farm or shop – meant that growing older would be associated with enhanced status and power. During that time, the structure of work was transformed; Irish people became employees, earning their livings in organisations on the basis of educational credentials (Breen *et al.*, 1990). Older people no longer possess the direct power over their children's lives which they formerly exercised, benevolently or otherwise, and age is no longer associated directly with power. The status of older people in Irish society remains unclear to this day.

Pensions were introduced in 1908 in tandem with those in England, and have mitigated the plights of older people without economic security, who – contrary to popular mythology – might be at considerable risk in the Ireland of those times. But pensions may not affect older people's well-being wholly beneficially. Phillipson (1993) is not alone in arguing that the notion of retirement has contributed to the social interpretation of ageing as a time of uselessness and irrelevance. It is true that widespread commitment to older people as a 'good cause' persists throughout Europe (Kohli, 1994), and also that older people in Ireland remain, until now, comparatively well protected in economic terms (Breen *et al.*, 1990: 96–7), though significant sub-groups form exceptions. But the nature of work in industrial societies is now in the process of renewed change, and the nature of ageing will change with it. Because of the profound nature of current economic transformations, and because developments in ageing include both radical improvements and radical threats, Ireland genuinely stands at a crossroads: ageing as a social and personal process may alter for the worse in future, or for the better.

This chapter will begin by discussing salient theoretical and empirical aspects of ageing in the contemporary Western world, treating ageing as a physical, social and personal process. In going on to deal with Ireland specifically, it will point to both the opportunities and the problems in our present situation, dealing first with health and well-being directly, and then with indicators of social support for well-being in older age such as community care, residential home provision and pensions policy. Issues related to family and gender are treated next, leading to conclusions about the conditions under which Irish people are currently constructing their life courses. In all these stages, both dangers and advantages affecting ageing will be underlined, illustrating the urgent nature of the case about which social and political decisions need to be made.

It is common to begin work on ageing by referring to numbers and proportions of 'older people' in the society concerned, but this practice should be regarded with caution. 'Older people' are often treated as a group including everyone over 65, but real ageing processes fluctuate considerably in type and timing; moreover, *highlighting* numerical information is in practice difficult to dissociate from the implication that older people form a threat to society *by virtue of* their numbers. Styles of reporting about ageing in themselves affect the way in which people conceive of ageing itself (cf. Edmondson, 1984). Conceptions of ageing are currently in flux as ageing itself changes; 'ageing' is not a potentially pathological state which strikes at 65, but develops differently, with different effects, throughout the life-course.

Forms of human maturation have been revolutionised over the last century; changes in nutrition, hygiene, housing and (perhaps to a lesser extent) medicine have meant that death is now much likelier to occur in later years than in infancy. For the first time in history, as Olshansky *et al.* emphasise (1993), the human mortality curve has diverged from the pattern common to all mammals, in which the first months and years of life are those where death is commonest. Our formerly pyramidal mortality curve is approaching the shape of a rectangle. The physical processes involved in ageing are imperfectly understood (Victor, 1994: 2ff.); hypotheses differ in their implications about the extent to which effects until now associated with ageing are modifiable. But if we are unclear about ageing in physical terms, we are even more unclear about it as a personal and social process, and emphasising numbers in a society of those defined as 'older' can render this confusion deeper. Laying stress on numbers by themselves makes it hard not to perceive older people as a static, homogeneous group, even while in principle we might realise they are not. This is not an argument against studying older age in terms which are partly quantitative, but it should alert us to possible side-effects of doing so.

Growing older takes different forms, for individuals and for social groups, according to the settings in which they find themselves. In any given society at any given time, there are groups of people moving through life in separate social, political and economic circumstances. Those born at approximately the same period, say within a decade, will encounter their own overall circumstances *as* a cohort – for instance war, depression, or economic recovery – but they will also differ, often spectacularly, *within* the cohort – according to gender, class, region and so on. Hence ageing is associated with different opportunities and constraints for each subgroup as it moves through time.

There are now relatively wealthy subgroups of (often male) older people in Europe who have benefited from advantageous occupational pension arrangements in the two or three decades of economic recovery following World War II – and whose 'oldness' itself takes a specific form. At the same time, there are extremely disadvantaged subgroups made up of those who happened to find themselves, at the relevant periods of their lives, in both cohort and socioeconomic positions to which these benefits did not apply. This shows that ageing is strongly affected, in practical terms, by changing societal developments; growing older does not bring with it the same benefits and the same disadvantages for everyone. In the Ireland which existed before the 1960s, social power on a local level attached to possessing property, and property tended to be concentrated in the hands of older owners, whose status was therefore improved by ageing; but for those falling outside this category, there is no reason to suppose that ageing presented at all the same advantages.

The nature of growing older is also affected by the way in which societies, or subcultures within societies, *regard* ageing. It is not a matter of 'mere' perception but of *practicality* that social expectations open or close avenues of conduct for those they affect. If, as happens increasingly often, in Ireland as elsewhere, it is expected that people are inappropriate candidates for new employment after they reach their forties, then individuals' own self-images in connection with ageing may be of little practical relevance: prevailing social preconceptions will ensure that they fail to get work. This is especially significant for women: if they have spent time raising children, then hope to resume their careers, public assumptions about ageing may detract from their chances of doing so. This problem is compounded by current increasingly fragmented career-structures. The demand that individuals accrue 'portfolios of skills' to be redeployed in different employment settings throughout their lives is plainly incompatible with employers' reluctance to take on 'middle-aged' workers. What 'ageing' means, and how the later stages of life-course construction can conduce to health and well-being for both individuals and societies, are therefore questions which have not yet been settled.

Ageing, Health and Well-being in Ireland

It is becoming accepted that good health should be understood in terms of a wide spectrum of forms of well-being (Kelleher, 1993), as a resource for creative use, rather than as a narrowly-conceived biomedical state. Increasing age is not necessarily associated with ill-health in the narrower interpretation, however. In Ireland as in Europe as a whole, the majority of older people lead independent lives; most care is self-care, followed by care by a spouse, then by some other family member (Eurobarometer, 1993). The fact that so much infirmity has retreated to later years is a triumph for contemporary forms of life-course construction, but it presents problems for those in later age-groups, not only directly but also indirectly, when they become perceived as making excessive claims on the social system. Negative social constructions such as this – which go so far as to cause allegations of 'generation war' in America – are illustrated in a newspaper report representing a prominent surgeon as suggesting that younger people with children should not be made to 'bear the financial burden' of health insurance for responding to illness in old age: '. . . the youth will not continue to pay up' (*Sunday Independent*, 2.2.1997). An alternative approach would see current younger cohorts as *advantaged* by relief from the ill-health borne by earlier generations, rather than disadvantaged by insurance contributions which will, in their own later years, benefit themselves.

The same report attributes alarm to the speaker because numbers of older people in Ireland may increase in future; this expectation must be seen in context. Fahey and Murray point out that while the number of older people in Ireland has increased this century, their proportion has remained similar, with 9.1% over 65 in 1926 and 11.4% in 1991. This compares with some 15% in Europe, where proportions are expected to rise to 20% in the next century (1994: 54–5). The survival rate of Irish people over 80 is expected to rise; there are currently more older women than men, a situation which may not continue (see below), and more older people in the West of Ireland – a disproportion which is expected to decrease, taking into account declines in agricultural employment and a consequent tendency for population to build up in the East (O'Shea, 1993: 16–17). Overall, in Ireland, a decline in the child population, a moderate increase in numbers of older people, and a rise in the working population (caused for instance by the entry of more women into the workforce) are together bringing about a *downward* trend in the 'dependency ratio' (Fahey and Murray, 1994: 60–1). Whether older people's increasing contribution to this ratio is associated with disproportionate expense in the future depends on ethical and political decisions as well as on *socially* related factors, including the salaries of medical personnel and the effects of health promotion on a wide range of preventable illnesses.

Although surviving to middle age is as common here as in other OECD countries, in Ireland 'life expectancy at older ages compares very poorly': the life expectancy of men 'has actually deteriorated over long periods during this century' (Fahey and Murray 1994: 13–20). As elsewhere, among older Irish people, there is a significant class and standard of living gradient in overall health, with poorer health in manual occupational groups and those suffering material deprivation (Fahey and Murray 1994: 16).

The health of people who are now older will have been affected by settings at earlier stages; 'cohort effects' combine with class effects to produce patterns of morbidity which are by no means all effects of ageing *per se*, so that the 'health status of older people' alters continuously.

As Fahey and Murray emphasise, ill-health in medical terms can severely detract from other capacities and pleasures – health in a wider sense. Although physical ill-health in older age is affected by events at earlier stages, this may in part be a social matter – for instance, when it is associated with work practices for which employers were responsible (Phillipson, 1993). Even 'lifestyle-related' behaviours known to produce ill-health later, such as smoking, almost certainly relate to aspects of social setting which are in principle modifiable. *Precisely how healthy* older age can become for entire populations cannot at present be known, given that widespread long-term survival is such a recent phenomenon. Utopianism in health care is currently distrusted, since the great twentieth-century welfare-state developments have not, for all their successes, effected the blanket transformations in health status anticipated from them. But reasons for this may be suggested; for example, the health improvements attendant on industrial society are also associated with new forms of stress and physical inactivity. Now, practices in mid-life have been identified which fundamentally enhance health and activity later (see, for example, Evans and Rosenberg, 1992); how widespread they become depends on individual and political decisions.

Health and well-being during different stages of life-course construction are influenced by social processes in a number of ways. On the one hand, older people may be being socialised to *expect* to be helpless, to underestimate their capacities (Walker, 1993); on the other hand, attitudes among medical person-nel to older people's health vary widely. In parts of North America, attitudes are much more proactive than in Ireland or Britain, where both medical practi-tioners and older people themselves often accept ill health as simply something to be endured (cf. Doress-Worters, Siegal *et al.*, 1994). The widespread assumption that all aspects of health must decline with age is incorrect, and may itself add to the psychological burden of physical complaints; Fahey and Murray report that psychological distress among their older respondents was often not caused by ageing *per se* but by illness and disability (1994: 18).

Health in the sense of well-being is also associated with features of societal structure unconnected with ageing as such – for instance, transport policy or social order. For example, almost a quarter of older respondents living alone in rural areas with no cars also have no access to any type of public transport (Fahey and Murray 1994: 17, 171). These are problems associated with low population density; in urban areas, by contrast, anxiety has been caused by increased experience of crime (Fahey and Murray 1994: 171). Thus, many problems perceived as connected with *ageing* are more properly analysed as problems *in society* to which ageing draws attention.

In keeping with the government policy document *The Years Ahead* (Department of Health, 1988), the eight Irish Health Boards approach support for older people in terms of 'community care'. The Eastern Health Board, for example, aims 'to maintain older people in dignity and independence at home' and 'to encourage and support the care of older people in their own community by family, neighbours and voluntary bodies'; it hopes 'to provide high quality hospital or residential care for older people' when this is not possible (1995: 1). About 5% of Irish older people live in some type of institution, though this proportion may rise in future (O'Shea and Hughes, 1994); it compares with a general European figure of between 3% and 6% (Victor, 1991: 25). Thus the community care approach corresponds in principle to the basic preference for independence attributable to many in the older population. In practice, however, its aims remain in large part aspirational, and exist in a setting of social attitudes to ageing which have not kept pace with contemporary developments in life-course construction.

Provisions for Successful Ageing

The Years Ahead stresses that older people should be enabled to live independently in communities with a wide spread of services to support their health and well-being. While there is increasing approval of such aims throughout Europe, experience shows that they are neither easy nor cheap to effect. Moreover, services are becoming increasingly fragmented, and the share contributed by the public sector is diminishing (O'Shea and Hughes, 1994: 176). This has different impacts throughout the sector; while there is a clear private market for residential care, for instance, there is less incentive for developing community care services privately. Provision of community centres and hospitals, with specialists in geriatric medicine, remains urgently in need of expansion (O'Shea *et al.*, 1991: 12–13).

Besides this, in Ireland, in the context of patchy overall provision, measures tend to be directed towards sections of the population who are perceived as vulnerable, needy or down-and-out. There is little sense of public, practical support for successful ageing as a normative expectation – although those measures which are in force, such as free travel passes, have a positive impact. In other settings (in parts of Bavaria, for example), a start has been made towards directing ageing policies towards positive enablement as such. Older people who *also happen to have* problems connected with health, poverty or social disability are assisted by the services relevant to those issues, so that neediness is not associated with ageing itself. In Ireland (as in Britain), community services, seeing themselves as responding to urgent *problems connected with ageing*, are drifting towards a residualist political philosophy. Older people are expected to look after themselves in the normal course of events. If they come into contact with public services it is because something is badly wrong with them; and, as on the nineteenth-century workhouse principle, some provisions are so uninviting that only a considerably disadvantaged person could feel comforted by them.

Public policy itself inevitably has a homogenising effect (Edmondson and Nullmeier, 1997); directing policy towards people makes it easier to perceive them as a single population, in .particular where providing 'care' is concerned. This is shown when, for instance, older people from contrasting social backgrounds are required to mix harmoniously in day-centres. However impeccable this expectation may be in principle, in practice it imposes considerable strain; older people who have struggled during their life-courses to improve their status, as they see it, may be utterly disconcerted when public policy reclassifies them back to the positions from which they started. In such contexts, ageing comes to be seen both by providers and by recipients of assistance as a problem in itself. On an 'empowerment' or 'citizenship' model, by contrast, public services would offer creative individual support to later stages of life-course construction just as they may to earlier ones.

Socially significant side-effects can therefore stem from well-intentioned policies, affecting the practical possibilities which ageing provides. *The Years Ahead*, for instance, takes it as axiomatic that older people should be treated with 'respect'; but 'respect' is an attitude which often situates its objects as 'other', as separate and different from 'ourselves'. Types of respect free of this potentially dangerous attribute tend to be based around some joint activity or function, and it is precisely uncertain, at present, what such a function might be as far as older people are concerned (though the 'mentor' system fostered by the IDA is sometimes suggested as a beginning). 'Respect' is undermined by a culture centred on youth which denies the existence of life-tasks beyond the range of consumer power – even though there is some evidence (see, for instance, Elder, 1974) that people in industrial societies regret having contributed to such a culture when they themselves become older. To enhance positive opportunities in later life stages, designated community personnel need to be given responsibility for services for older people, as O'Shea *et al.* suggest (1991: 128), but these services should not be designed only to provide 'care'. They should also develop the status and cultural integration of older people.

Community care services currently available are irregular in extent; people in need of support often fail to get it. Lundström and McKeown report that the following response, from an older inhabitant in an urban region, is 'typical':

> The one [Public Health Nurse] that goes around here . . . she's inundated with work. She's all this locality for just one nurse. Yes, she's all this place, so I don't blame her in a way for not calling . . . she never calls near me (1994: 289).

These authors indicate that, in a complex and under-researched scenario in which even official data-collection is inadequate, obtaining assistance such as home help can be simply a matter of luck. Many regions of the country depend heavily on voluntary services, and overall cost-efficiency is achieved by 'considerably less expenditure on staff salaries, inferior conditions of employment and a lack of investment in training' (1994: 297). It is not even agreed what home helps are for (Lundström and McKeown: 305): should they provide practical aid or personal and psychological support? Home helps themselves are a vulnerable group; the worst paid, in the West, are remunerated at the rate of £1 an hour. Similarly, paramedical services in the community 'are negligible (and not much better in institutions)' (O'Shea *et al.*, 1991: 45). The official aim of 'community care' is to enhance the independence of older people, but there is as yet no systematic approach to achieving this in practice. Ireland's eight Regional Health Boards have very different approaches to conceptualising and funding it (Lundström and McKeown, 1994): cost, payment, the nature of care and who provides it all fluctuate between areas.

The Eurobarometer indicates, however, that high proportions of individuals across Europe regularly provide support to older family and friends (1993), and there is evidence that many enjoy doing so. In Ireland, the public services are claimed to provide some 9% of all care, as against 25% in Britain (Victor, 1994); Blackwell *et al.* (1992) report that the majority of private 'carers' are female and themselves not young, with an average age of 52 years; for women like this, the opportunity cost of caring may increase in future generations. Only a minority of full-time carers now receive any financial support; extending this, as well for example as day-centre provisions, could lead to a reduction in the need for costly institutional care in the future (O'Shea, 1993: 85). But even the term 'care' may affect those who give and receive it, since 'care', like 'old age' itself, tends to become a stigmatising 'master concept' defining the entire situation of anyone involved. An experienced farmer or company director with a broken hip is transformed, perhaps overnight, by becoming a 'recipient of care' and his or her spouse a 'carer'. Attention to the needs of people who give wholesale support to others is essential if private support is not to be treated as a cheap alternative to public care; but it should not entail blanket conceptualisations of 'carers' or recipients of 'care'.

As far as residential provisions for older people are concerned, O'Shea *et al.* point out that considerable growth has occurred as 'a relatively silent phenomenon', independent of policy decisions and generated largely privately (1991: 7). In three years, between 1986 and 1989, the number of private nursing homes in the Eastern region grew by 115% (O'Shea *et al.*, 1991: 31–3). Residential homes tend to be small private enterprises, and there is little evidence that many are conceived around positive models of ageing. Most often, residents sleep in shared or single bedrooms and spend the daytime in common-rooms, seldom engaging in significant activity (cf. M. O'Shea, 1993). Little or no 'occupational therapy' is commonly available, let alone any route to genuine contribution to worthwhile tasks. O'Connor and Thompstone (1986) suggest that 'homes' tend to maintain dependence rather than independence, with no structures in place to allow residents to maintain links with any other part of the community.

This does not mean that individual homes are not doing their best according to their lights, rather that there is a deficit in *societal* expectations of what should be aspired to in terms of spending later life stages. A wider variety of retirement homes could extend independent living rather than 'care'; different types of sheltered housing and retirement community are now appearing and will probably increase in number, but they are likely to be relatively expensive (O'Connor *et al.*, 1989). Some areas, such as the West, appear particularly deficient in provisions; many of the most creative depend on voluntary organisations like 'Share' in Cork. The 1990 Health (Nursing Homes) Act introduces a system of registration but does not lay down an obligatory code of practice. Such a code could usefully be overseen by a central body in future, offering arrangements making complaints practicable, with a presumption in favour both of residents contacting advocate organisations, and of contributing to communal life much more effectively than is currently possible.

At present, people are more likely to enter institutions if they cannot live with family or friends, or if community supports are inadequate; that is, social as well as medical reasons contribute heavily to individuals' entry into residential homes. Moreover, there is danger that a two-tier system is developing, with less well-resourced individuals living in 'relatively spartan conditions' (O'Shea *et al.*, 1991: 14). To combat invidious distinctions, O'Shea *et al.* (1991: 34ff.) recommend that financing for residential care should be administered on social insurance principles, across the entire population. This would ensure earmarked funds for everyone as they get older, protecting against the attrition which is likely to ensue as governments in the future continue to be concerned about mounting numbers of older people.

Other forms of financing residential care can have drastic effects on lifecourse construction as a general social process, not just on the individuals immediately affected. Funding which is linked to the sale of housing, for instance, undermines a powerful social symbol for the unity and purpose of individual and family life – not to mention practical difficulties if only one of a family needs institutional care, or if someone is placed in a residential home but wishes to leave. Some 75% of heads of household over 65 in Ireland own their houses outright, but they are not necessarily wealthy: 58% of owners have disposable income in the lowest three deciles (Callan *et al.*, 1989). The houses in question are not all of high market value; but in an Irish context, owning a home indicates life-course well-being (see also O'Shea *et al.*, 1991: 30). Selling people's homes retrospectively undermines a central source of personal validity for their owners, and may have a negative effect on social order by casting general doubt over the permanence of symbols of life-course construction.

'Old age' is often officially defined in terms of retirement, but the pension may not be simply a straightforward improvement in conditions for well-being. Pensions have saved many people from the fear of destitution (see O'Shea, 1993: ch.2); but in the context of a work-oriented, youth-oriented society they also create an image of older people as debarred from the mainstream of life. Whelan and Whelan (1988) show that, in Ireland as elsewhere, actual retirement ages are now scattered widely; only a quarter of their respondents retired at 65. The many possible reasons for early retirement – which usually entails considerable financial penalties – include restructuring, disguising unemployment (Guillemard, 1986), and changing attitudes to work, as well as ill-health, caused by working conditions or otherwise. Being retired, being over 65, and being 'old' are no longer synonymous: the 1996 Inbucon report (1996: 78) locates 'normal' early retirement among executives between 50 and 55.

The question of pensions, then, illustrates contemporary changes in ageing and perceiving ageing.[1] Not all these changes are liberating; the advantages of giving individuals main responsibility for directing their life-courses diminish within a setting dominated by vastly more powerful players. As work-structures fragment, occupational pension arrangements increasingly become individuals' own responsibility; but most people do not take the attitudes to their own life-courses which would enable them to devise pensions effectively. They do not appear to regard their own lives as planned projects (cf. Connolly, 1991); frequently, they do not initiate pension payments early enough, and may be too preoccupied with predicaments characteristic of earlier life-course stages to be able to do so. Even the most pragmatic and inventive individuals more often expect to *respond to* life circumstances than to shape them in their entirety, and all are faced with three powerful sources of uncertainty: the incalculability of the employment structure, the complexity of the private pensions market (and the misinformation sometimes associated with it), together with governments' capacity to legislate to alter pension provisions in retrospect. If life-course construction is to become a personal project, the example of pension provision illustrates the fact that it also needs strong political defences.

Family, Gender and Life-Course Construction

In industrial societies, practical and financial assistance tends to travel *from* older generations towards younger ones, rather than the other way round (Finch, 1989). This contrasts with the patterns rural Ireland used to exhibit, where children provided considerable assistance in farm work (Curtin and Varley, 1984), and younger people played a markedly subordinate role in the division of responsibilities between generations; even adult children were not expected to contradict their elders. An early sociological portrayal of older people's lives in Ireland, by Arensberg and Kimball, sees the Ireland of the 1930s as 'in some ways an old person's country' (1940: 158). They argue that older people of the time 'are honored. They have power' (1940: 167–8). Unsurprisingly, Irish respondents for the 1993 Eurobarometer reported experiencing more respect as they grew older; in the nature of the case, their status as adults is likely to be higher than it was when they were children.

Close familial relations between generations in the past were dictated by economic considerations in the first place, and did not necessarily run by any means smoothly (Brown, 1985: ch.2); household sizes are now declining, which may sometimes enhance relationships. Ten per cent of the Irish population lived alone in 1961 and 21% in 1986; in other OECD countries, the level is 40% (O'Shea, 1993: 39). For most people now older, family relations remain central to their lives, but families themselves have changed during their life-times. Childhood dependence now lasts longer, and includes extensive periods of education; married couples may survive for half a century together (Vincent, 1995: 160). In consequence of these changes, older people live in several social worlds simultaneously, following some expectations stemming from their youth and others from different life-stages. Fahey and Murray report that over 80% of their women respondents say they never go out for a drink, but most of the men do (1994: 82). On the other hand, although married women now in their seventies were usually not expected to obtain professions when they were younger, they may apply different standards when they look back on their lives now.

Though the implications of personal attitudes for well-being may be commonly admitted, their roots in social systems and political economies are often ignored. For example, attention is given both in policy-making and in popular imagination to problems with 'loneliness' in older age, despite conflicting information about its extent; however, loneliness is probably not one phenomenon but several, with different structural causes. Townsend (1957) suggests that loneliness may result from traumatic experiences such as the death of intimates, rather than from simple lack of interaction with other human beings – whose value to different groups of older people we do not yet understand: Pat O'Connor's work (1994) shows that relationships can be interpreted differently by the very people engaged in them. Fahey and Murray report interaction with neighbours to be as frequent as that with family in Ireland (1994: 118), but we know little about the felt significance this has. In any case, concentrating analysis on problems perceived as personal distracts from systemic questions about the roles possible in later stages of life-construction; significant types of 'loneliness' may be connected with lack of meaningful social participation, or with lack of social power.

Older people may be excluded from power structures by expectations that their life-stages are no longer interesting. Women may also be excluded from these structures by other aspects of life-course conventions, which fail to recognise that parents with the main responsibility for children have different life-course structures from people who have none. This has adverse effects on women's careers, for it is not usual for either qualification levels or pension rights to take account of time spent child-rearing. Child-bearing stages tend to be treated, from the standpoint of careers, pensions, and the perception of appropriate timing for professional activities, as a private self-indulgence. Age discrimination itself 'is not an issue that has received much attention in Ireland' (O'Shea, 1993: 58); when this changes, its gender-related aspects should be to the fore.

At present, women run a greater risk of poverty in old age than men (O'Shea, 1993); because of their current longer longevity they also stand a greater chance of living alone. This will not necessarily persist; women have lived longer in this century only, as a result of factors such as improved medical hygiene at childbirth. If the social behaviour of the genders continues to coincide, so may their lengths of life. Both now die most often from circulatory diseases and cancers. Two thirds of Ireland's population aged 65 or over report that they are in good health, but women have more functional incapacity at all ages, and particularly as they grow older (Fahey and Murray, 1994: 186, 86–7). For men, by contrast, old age may be 'the most relaxed, distress-free stage of life' (1994: 93) – perhaps partly because they have left the world of work.[2] The life satisfactions versus the tensions which each gender derives from work need further comparison; if, in the past, many women worked mainly to escape social isolation (Byrne *et al.*, 1995), ceasing work may affect their old age differently, intensifying isolation rather than freeing from stress.

Women are currently those most often responsible for 'care' given to older family members. 'Caring' is of different types, ranging up to a 24-hour presence (O'Connor *et al.*, 1988); care of people with Alzheimer's disease is uniquely stressful and gruelling. Critics of community care argue that, in effect, it shifts care from the State's responsibility to that of women, whose own health and well-being may be drastically affected (see Dalley, 1988). There are radical discrepancies between career-related expectations applied to women and the care functions demanded of them, particularly for women who finish caring for their children just as their parents begin to require care. Moreover, these women cannot rely on reciprocal contributions for themselves later, for their children's conception of how to construct a life-course is changing; what old age will hold for them cannot yet be known.

Approaches to Life-Course Construction in an Irish Context

Theories of ageing differ, first, according to whether they emphasise interacting social *processes* in a dynamic fashion, or whether they reify older people as a separate social *group*. Secondly, some theories are methodological, directing us *where to look* to explore life-course construction, and others are substantive, attributing particular *contents* to the latter stages of people's lives. Though adhering to the first of each pair may be preferable, it is not fail-safe by itself, as the widely disparaged 'disengagement theory' illustrates (Cumming and Henry, 1961). Taking a functionalist approach, their research asserts that older people retreat contentedly from engagement in social processes in order to make way for new generations. This work is now seen as inferring from an untypical sample, under the unconscious influence of an ideology *wishing* older people to fade away without fuss or expense.

Research like this has led to a preoccupation in critical gerontology with the insidiousness with which work on older people reflects discriminatory assumptions. Methodological theories which make special efforts to avoid this include life-course centred approaches whose accounts of setting emphasise competition for resources of power and money (cf. Dant, 1988), competition which contributes to an evolving cultural landscape in which it is possible to become one kind of person more easily than another. This combines Hareven's emphasis on life-courses and the different timings they may involve (1977) with the 'political economy' approach. From this standpoint, Walker (1993) points to the contemporary ideological hegemony pressurising older people themselves into believing that they constitute a problem; Phillipson (1993) argues that the consumerist culture which succeeded World War II has obstructed us from evolving creative forms of ageing to suit current contexts.

Intentionally or otherwise, most theories of ageing have normative implications; here sociological theories need to respond to psychological accounts stressing possibilities of development at all stages of the life course (Erikson *et al.*, 1986). But where Havighurst's 'activity theory' (1963) has been claimed to urge older people to ignore ageing altogether, the Rileys (1986) recommend a return to Aristotle. According to him, one's true potential as a human being can be defined by the way in which one spends one's leisure time. The middle-aged, according to this position, are enslaved to the world of work; older people are those with the opportunity to evolve a culture which establishes genuine goals for life in society (Wörner, 1997). This approach, like those of Young and Schuller (1991) and Laslett (1992), insists that new forms of ageing require new analyses of what life-course construction could and should contain. It insists that the positive, rather than the negative, potential in contemporary ageing should be developed and embraced.

To understand processes of life-course construction in Ireland from the viewpoints of participants, to discover what ageing is actually like as a social experience, it will be necessary to track different approaches to building up a life among different sections of the population. This cannot be done without a long-term, hermeneutic approach to exploring meaning, since many forms of academic data-collection fail to respond to the communicative forms used by older people themselves (Edmondson, 1995). Far from being easily formulable in brief interaction with strangers, attitudes related to health, ageing and well-being may be best or only expressible indirectly; it is unlikely that they can be elicited effectively by methods which rely on seeking direct propositions about respondents' inner worlds. Attitudes are not just cognitive items in respondents' minds which can be reported on; they form aspects of *practices*, parts of living lives. Meaning is often only perceptible to either actor or observer as a consequence of *sequences* of interaction; methods for discovering attitudes affecting life-course construction will often require processes of interaction as well as consultation with respondents themselves.

In Ireland, longitudinal studies with strong qualitative aspects will therefore be needed to track developments within a social system where ageing as a process is changing, and within which there are considerable weaknesses in provision. Central recommendations of *The Years Ahead* for community care still have not been implemented. Both individual and institutional abuse of older people, which may have many causes and may take many forms – physical, psychological, social and legal – needs to be better understood (Madden, 1992). At present, there is little opportunity for vulnerable sections of the older population even to make their experiences known, and the extent of this problem is under-explored. Thus, while older people in Ireland enjoy some overall advantages, such as those in fiscal terms, major challenges surround developing these within new patterns of life-course construction, and responding to the demands of genuine community care.

Public policy is currently constructed under circumstances of some ignorance about the outcomes of different kinds of support (O'Shea *et al.* 1991: 27). We need to discover much more about how older age can be spent constructively. Appropriate research should be self-critical and reflexive, since theories related to health and care are highly vulnerable to intellectual fashion. Just as the Victorians took it for granted that large-scale approaches to health problems would be optimal, nowadays individualist, activist solutions possess automatic appeal; but they risk ignoring social effects and social needs, imposing solutions from outside the changing positions occupied by older people themselves. We need, therefore, to develop ways in which older people can contribute their own decisions to both the private and the public processes which affect them, and to facilitate their cultural and economic integration into areas of society where they wish to belong. It is hard to see that life-course construction can be improved for anyone if we segregate part of the population as 'old'; both theory and practice should explore the full social and individual benefits to be derived from all stages of the life course.

Notes

The research which this article is connected was funded by the Health Research Board in conjunction with the Centre for Health Promotion Studies, University College, Galway.

1   Pension policy is a central issue in highlighting the interplay of positive and negative developments in opportunities for well-being in older age – 'health' as envisaged by the World Health Organisation – as these developments are influenced by a conjunction of socioeconomic, cultural and political factors. It is thus a central feature for consideration in sociological approaches to ageing. For a more strictly epidemiological approach to morbidity and mortality in Ireland this century, see for example Shelley, 1995.
2   This finding by Fahey and Murray is striking and unusual: it points to the need for expanded research on the connection between health, as broadly conceived, and the experience of work in Ireland. We do not know, for example, what sort of work these respondents have left – for example, how much of it it resembles older- or newer-style work patterns – so we do not know exactly what this finding points to for the future.

References

Arensberg, Conrad and Solon Kimball (1940) *Family and Community in Ireland.* Cambridge, Mass: Harvard University Press.

Bond, John, Peter Coleman and Sheila Peace (eds) (1993) *Ageing in Society: An Introduction to Social Gerontology.* London: Sage.

Blackwell, John, E. O'Shea, G. Moane and P. Murray (1992) *Care Provision and Cost Measurement: Dependent Elderly People at Home and in Geriatric Hospitals.* Dublin: Economic and Social Research Institute.

Breen, Richard, Damian Hanan, David Rottman and Christopher Whelan (1990) *Understanding Contemporary Ireland.* Houndmills: Macmillan.

Brown, Terence (1985) *Ireland: A Social and Cultural History* (2nd edn). London: Fontana.

Byrne, Anne, Mary Owens, Breda Lymer and Catherine Conlon (1995) *Republic of Ireland National Report: Rural Women's Research Project.* Galway: UCG Women's Studies Centre.

Callan T., D.F. Hannan, B. Nolan, B. J. Whelan and S. Creighton (1989) *The Measurement of Poverty and Social Welfare Effectiveness in Ireland.* Dublin: Economic and Social Research Institute.

Connolly, William E. (1991) *Identity/Difference. Democratic Negotiations of Political Paradox.* Ithaca: Cornell University Press.

Cumming, E. and W. Henry (1961) *Growing Old: The Process of Disengagement.* New York: Basic Books.

Curtin, Chris and Tony Varley (1984) Children and childhood in rural Ireland, in: Chris Curtin, Mary Kelly and Liam O'Dowd (eds), *Culture and Ideology in Ireland.* Galway: Galway University Press: 30–45.

Dalley, Gillian (1988) *Ideologies of Caring.* Houndmills: Macmillan.

Dant, T., 1988. Dependency and old age: theoretical accounts and practical understandings, *Ageing and Society:* 171–88.

Department of Health (1988) *The Years Ahead: A Report of the Working Party on Services for the Elderly.* Dublin: GPSO.

Doress-Worters, Paula, Diana Laskin Siegal and the Boston Women's Health Book Collective (1994) *The New Ourselves Growing Older* (2nd edn). New York: Simon and Schuster.

Eastern Health Board (1995) *Review of Services for the Elderly and Four-Year Action Plan 1995–1998*. Dublin.

Edmondson, Ricca (1995a) *Rhetoric in Sociology*. London: Macmillan.

Edmondson, Ricca (1995b) Critical ethnography and policy on ageing in: George Taylor (ed.), *Centre for Public Policy Working Papers*. Galway: Social Sciences Research Centre.

Edmondson, Ricca (1997) Silence and the golden years: older people and social policy in Ireland, in: George Taylor (ed.), *The Politics of Irish Public Policy*. Galway: UCG Press.

Edmondson, Ricca and Frank Nullmeier (1997) Knowledge and rhetoric as Contexts for Political Action, in R. Edmondson (ed.), *The Political Context of Collective Action: Argumentation, Power and Democracy*. London: Routledge.

Elder, Glen (1974) *Children of the Great Depression: Social Change in Life Experience*. Chicago: University of Chicago Press.

Erikson, E.H, J.M. Erikson and H.Q. Kivnick (1986) *Vital Involvement in Old Age: the Experience of Old Age in Our Time*. New York: Norton.

Evans, William and Irwin Rosenberg (1992) *Biomarkers*. New York: Simon & Schuster.

Eurobarometer (1993) *Age and Attitudes: Main Results of a Eurobarometer Survey*. Brussels: Directorate-General 5, European Commission.

Fahey, Tony and Peter Murray (1994) *Health and Autonomy Among the Over-65s in Ireland*. Dublin: National Council for the Elderly.

Finch, Janet (1989) *Family Obligations and Social Change*. Cambridge: Polity.

Guillemard, Anne-Marie (1986) Social policy and ageing in France, in: C. Phillipson and A. Walker (eds), *Ageing and Social Policy: A Critical Assesment*. London: Gower: 263–79.

Hareven, Tamara (1977) Family time and historical time, *Daedalus*, 106: 57–70.

Hareven, Tamara (1982) The life course and aging in historical perspective, in: T. Hareven and K. Adams (eds), *Ageing and Life Course Transitions: An Interdisciplinary Perspective*. London: Tavistock: 1–26.

Havighurst, R.J. (1963) Successful ageing in R.H. Williams, C. Tibbitts and W. Donahue (eds), *Processes of Ageing*, vol. I. New York: Atherton: 299–320.

Inbucon Ireland Ltd (1996) *Report on Executive Salaries and Fringe Benefits in Ireland, 1996*. Dublin: Inbucon.

Kelleher, Cecily (1993) *Measures to Promote Health and Autonomy for Older People: A Position Paper*. Dublin: National Council for the Elderly.

Kohli, Martin (1994) 'Solidarity between generations: from state back to market and the family'; Symposium Address to XIIIth World Congress of Sociology, Bielefeld.

Laslett, Peter (1992) *A Fresh Map of Life: the Emergence of the Third Age*. London: Weidenfeld and Nicholson.

Lundström, Francesca and Kieran McKeown (1994) *Home Help Services for Elderly People in Ireland*. Dublin: National Council for the Elderly.

Madden, Patrick (1992) Towards health promotion of the elderly, unpublished paper.

O'Connor, J. and K. Thompstone (1986) *Nursing Homes in the Republic of Ireland: A Study of the Private and Voluntary Sector*. Dublin: National Council for the Aged.

O'Connor, J., H. Ruddle, M. O'Gallagher and E. Murphy (1988) *The Caring Process: A Study of Carers in the Home*. Dublin: National Council for the Aged.

O'Connor, J., H. Ruddle and M. O'Gallagher (1989) *Sheltered Housing in Ireland: its Role and Contributions in the Care of the Elderly.* Dublin: National Council for the Aged.

O'Connor, Pat (1994) Very close parent–child relationships: the perspective of the elderly person, *Journal of Cross-Cultural Gerontology,* 9: 53–76.

Olshansky, Jay, Bruce Carnes and Christine Casall (1993) The aging of the human species, *Scientific American,* 268 (4): 46–52.

O'Shea, Eamon (1993) *The Impact of Social and Economic Policies on Older People in Ireland.* Dublin: National Council for the Elderly.

O'Shea, Eamon, David Donnison and Joe Larragy *et al.* (1991) *The Role and Future Development of Nursing Homes in Ireland.* Dublin: National Council for the Elderly.

O'Shea, Eamon and Jenny Hughes (1994) *The Economics and Financing of Long-term Care of the Elderly in Ireland.* Dublin: National Council for the Elderly.

O'Shea, Maura (1993) 'The contribution of private nursing homes to care of the elderly in County Galway', Galway: thesis for membership of the Faculty of Public Health Medicine in Ireland. ·

Phillipson, C. and A. Walker (eds) (1986) *Ageing and Social Policy: A Critical Assesment.* London: Gower.

Phillipson, Chris (1993) The sociology of retirement, in John Bond, Peter Coleman and Sheila Peace (eds), *Ageing in Society: An Introduction to Social Gerontology.* London: Sage: 180–99.

Riley, Martha and John Riley (1986) Longevity and social structure: the potential of the added years, in Alan Pfifer and Lydia Bronte (eds), *Our Aging Society: Paradox and Promise.* New York: Norton : 53–7.

Shelley, Emer (1995) *The Kilkenny Health Project Final Report.* Kilkenny: Kilkenny Health Project.

Townsend, Peter (1957) *The Family Life of Old People.* London: Routledge & Kegan Paul.

Victor, Christina (1991) *Health and Health Care in Later Life.* Buckingham: Open University Press.

Victor, Christina (1994) *Old Age in Modern Society* (2nd edition). London: Chapman and Hall.

Vincent, John (1995) *Inequality and Old Age.* London: UCL Press.

Walker, Alan (1993) Poverty and inequality in old age, in Bond *et al.* (eds), *Ageing in Society.* London: Sage: 280–303.

Whelan, C.T. and B.J. Whelan (1988) *The Transition to Retirement.* Dublin: Economic and Social Research Institute.

Wörner, Markus (1997) A culture of friendship: societal wellbeing and older age, in: M. Barry, R. Edmondson and C. Kelleher (eds), *Working Papers in the Theory of Health.* Galway: Social Sciences Research Centre.

Young, Michael and Tom Schuller (1991) *Life After Work: The Arrival of the Ageless Society.* London: Harper-Collins.

Section 4

MENTAL HEALTH

11

Alcoholism in Ireland

Tanya M. Cassidy

Despite popular belief, often propagated by groups such as Alcoholics Anonymous (AA), alcoholism is not a straightforward or simple topic to discuss. Almost since its inception the term has been contested. Discussing this topic in Ireland adds a further level of complexity to the discussion, one that brings into question stereotypes and their influences on individuals, practitioners and researchers. The belief that the Irish were particularly prone to alcoholism has often been accepted as a given. In fact, researchers such as Robert F. Bales argued that the Irish cultural drinking patterns represented the archetypal 'alcoholic addiction' (Bales, 1980[1944]; Bales, 1962; Pittman, 1967). In recent years this assumption has been debated, and the complexities of Irish drinking acknowledged. A recent Irish government publication stated that '[t]here is evidence that the description of the Irish as a particularly alcohol-prone race is a myth' (Department of Health, 1996: 11). This 'surprising finding' (in the words of the report) has been quietly noted for centuries, but has often been drowned out by contrary stereotypical descriptions. Furthermore, this myth or stereotypical belief has influenced many of the conclusions reached by numerous researchers on issues related to alcohol in Ireland (Cassidy, 1996; 1997).

Alcohol is a social drug which, to this day, evokes the divisive moral qualities that originated, or at least were solidified, in the last century with the birth of temperance movements. Temperance movements from the earliest days have appealed to 'scientific' or 'medical' disease models of alcohol-related problems. Among other problems, the modern world saw the emergence of alcohol addiction, later termed alcoholism, and most recently 'alcohol dependency syndrome'. Of course, problems related to alcohol existed prior to this age, but these problems were reconceptualised at the end of the eighteenth century, a time period in which a 'shift in gaze' occurred, according to Foucault (1967; 1977). In Ireland this time period is marked by changes in the drinks industry, particularly for distilled beverages. Furthermore, this time period is also marked by the popularisation, particularly in England, of the stereotypical image of a whiskey-drinking Irishman. This image was to be further entrenched in Irish society with the birth of Father Mathew's temperance crusade, the legacy of which still reverberates through Irish society. The large percentage of people who have never drunk alcohol in their lives is largely attributed to the Pioneer Total Abstinence Association.

Three main indices used to measure, and compare, national levels of 'alcoholism' are discussed: cirrhosis of the liver mortality rates, national alcohol consumption rates, and hospitalisation rates for diagnoses related to alcohol. Over the years, each of these measures has been subjected to extensive criticisms, resulting in increased use of survey methods, and a recognition of the importance of more individual-level characteristics. Very recently, Single (1995) has argued that we should be considering the number of heavy drinking occasions, rather than overall consumption rates, in an attempt to reduce the harmful effects of alcohol. This vision is informed by research which suggests that both ends of the drinking continuum (heavy consumption and total abstinence) lead to health problems. It has been argued that moderate consumption of alcohol is not only advisable, but actually healthy (Renaud and de Lorgeril, 1992; Gronbaek *et al.*, 1994). These recent conclusions have begun to have wide-ranging treatment and policy implications.

Socio-Historical Notions Surrounding Alcohol and Health

Alcoholism is defined in the Oxford English Dictionary (OED) to be '[t]he action of alcohol upon the human system; diseased condition produced by alcohol' (1933: 210), which seems to imply the notion that anyone can be affected by this 'diseased condition'. On the other hand, the American definition from Merriam-Webster defines alcoholism as 'a complex chronic psychological and nutritional disorder associated with excessive and usually compulsive drinking' (1989: 69). This definition implies that only certain people might become affected by alcoholism, particularly individuals who drink heavily. At the heart of these two definitions is the underlying moral debate that has plagued the study of alcohol issues at least throughout this century.

The term 'alcoholism' is relatively modern, dating to the mid-nineteenth century.[1] It was first introduced in 1852 by Dr Magnus Huss of Stockholm, who used it to refer to a special chronic condition of 'inebriates' (the preferred term in the nineteenth century). As Keller said, 'the world had needed the right word for It, and alcoholism was it' (1982: 121). By 1869 the *Daily News* (8 December) reports 'the deaths of 2 persons from alcoholism'[2] (OED, 1933: 210). 'The word' as Keller points out, 'became common' (1982: 123).

Doctor Huss' Latin-Swedish neologism passed into everyday international speech and thereby experienced the fate of many ordinary words: It was made more and more useful. Its meaning was popularly enriched—and thereby technically impoverished. It ceased to be solely a diagnostic term for a condition identified by specifiable symptoms. And popular usage is not without influence on professionals (Keller, 1982: 123).

As time progressed the term alcoholism began to take on broader meanings; Keller points out that 'in the first *Dictionary of Words about Alcohol* (1968), many pages were devoted to the definition of alcoholism and cognate terms' (1982: 119). In fact, over the years '[m]any many writers felt a need to formulate their own definitions' (Keller, 1982: 119). It is for this reason, Keller argues, that the term 'alcoholism' became such a contested concept, leading to its disfavour in research circles. The rise and eventual demise of the term 'alcoholism', is not the topic of this paper (see Cassidy, 1997); suffice it to say that the term is now mainly used by lay people and some medical professionals.[3] This does not mean that issues related to health and alcohol have been disregarded; on the contrary, many of the same debates continue, although researchers now discuss 'alcohol problems', and medical practitioners discuss 'alcohol dependency syndrome' which harkens back to the pre-alcoholism notions of addiction.

Alcohol issues were 'medicalised' well before the emergence of the term alcoholism, and were originally tied to notions of addiction. The famous eighteenth-century American physician, Benjamin Rush, could be described as the 'Father of Medicalising Alcohol Issues'. As Levine (1978) has pointed out, the concept of alcohol addiction was first clearly developed in the works of Benjamin Rush (1785) and later was to become intimately linked to issues of temperance. Specifically, Rush saw the 'disease of inebriety' as a 'disease of the will' which researchers have pointed out was 'based on the then popular assumption that one's "will" and "desire" were quite distinct' (Conrad and Schneider, 1980: 81). He believed that the 'disease of inebriety', was caused by an 'addiction' to alcohol, particularly spirits, due to long-term excessive use.

> It belongs to the history of drunkenness to remark, that its paroxysms occur, like the paroxysms of many diseases, at certain periods, and after longer or shorter intervals. They often begin with annual, and gradually increase in their frequency, until they appear in quarterly, monthly, weekly, and quotidian or daily periods (Rush, 1943[1785]: 192).

In many ways, Rush's vision of alcohol-related problems saw the source or root being the alcohol itself. Potentially, anyone who consumed this product, in particular the most dangerous and vulgar distilled versions, could succumb to this believed-to-be progressive disease. Thus it is not surprising that Rush's arguments were taken on by many early temperance campaigners, the earliest of whom were chiefly anti-spirits.

Meanwhile in Britain, a similar, but less philosophical, vision was being put forth by Thomas Trotter. In 1788, Trotter wrote, as partial requirement for a medical degree at the University of Edinburgh, that 'the habit of drunkenness is a disease of the mind' (1941[1804]: 586).

> This disease, I mean the habit of drunkenness, is like some other mental derangements; there is an ascendancy to be gained over the person committed to our care, which, when accomplished, brings him entirely under our control. (Trotter, 1941[1804]: 586–7).

Trotter and other English and European colleagues saw themselves as prescribing a more 'scientific' approach, and thus avoided traditional moral language, no longer speaking of the drunkard's 'love' of drink, but rather talking about physiological conditions of 'craving' and 'insatiable desire'. The problem and resultant solution for the European analysts were seen to lie not in drink, but in the drinker. However, like Rush, the first and foremost step in treatment was seen to be total abstinence from all alcoholic beverages.

Irish Drunkenness from Sin to Sickness

The late eighteenth century and early nineteenth century in Ireland were marked by an anti-whiskey campaign among the Protestant Ascendancy; like so much of Irish history, this was intimately tied to sectarian divisions. The distilling and brewing industries were divided by religion: distilling was dominated by Catholics, while the more expensive commercial brewing industry was dominated by wealthy Protestants. Furthermore, legislation was also introduced at this time which regulated the production of distilled beverages, resulting in the closure of many distilleries throughout Ireland. Coinciding with these anti-whiskey legislative changes were others that favoured brewed beverages, and so contributed to the growth and expansion of the brewing industry. Many of these 'enlightened' wealthy had numerous reasons to advocate the consumption of brewed beverages, and argued that the consumption of distilled spirits caused, or at least exacerbated, poverty among the lower classes (Bretherton, 1991). Like similar campaigns at the same time in other countries,[4] this early temperance movement was not anti-alcohol per se, but rather anti-spirits. The poor were encouraged to make brewed beverages their preferred choice of intoxicant, whereas the upper classes continued to enjoy such beverages as wine and/or brandy.

This early campaign became linked to Protestantism and failed to enlist any substantial part of the vast Catholic population. In fact, as Maguire says in an early biography of Father Mathew, many were suspicious of this early temperance movement as an attempt 'on the part of Protestants "to entangle Catholics in their society"' (1863: 101). Even Bishop James Doyle, the only member of the Catholic hierarchy who supported this early Protestant temperance movement, doubted its success. In a letter in 1829, he said 'I am not prepared to express to others a confidence which I do not feel, that such societies in this country at this time, with our present laws and social government, can be productive of any great, or extensive, or permanent good' (Malcolm, 1986: 84).

Things were to change dramatically with the advent of the second wave of temperance supporters. In the 1830s, anti-alcohol sentiments were to harden, as they had in many other countries, to advocating total abstinence (Bretherton, 1991). This seems to have been spearheaded by people of humbler means who saw the earlier paternalistic movement of the Protestant ascendancy as hypocritical, and designed to allow the rich to continue to enjoy their wine. This new wave, however, was also mainly associated with Protestants, and did not spread to Catholics until 1838 when William Martin, a Quaker who founded the Cork Total Abstinence Society three years earlier, enlisted the help of Father Theobald Mathew.

Enlisting a Catholic priest gave credence to the movement for the majority of the Irish population, and it quickly spread. It was, as Kerrigan said, 'inevitable' that the temperance movement would become linked to O'Connell's repeal campaign, 'given that both found their support, or most of it, among the Catholic population' (1992: 107). This linkage began in 1839 when O'Connell gave a speech in Bandon, Cork, where he linked temperance to increased wealth for the nation and political change (Malcolm, 1986: 128; Kerrigan, 1992: 107). In the following year, the Reverend James Birmingham said

> Ireland should stand still or retrograde, until the foul stigma had been wiped off, which the habitual intemperance of her sons cast upon her. And, in truth, not only were our countrymen remarkable for the intemperate use of intoxicating liquors, but intemperance had already entered into, and formed a part of the national character. An Irishman and a drunkard had become synonymous terms . . . and a frequent, if not a strictly just argument set up against our claims for liberty was, that a people so enslaved to a base and demoralising habit, could not be entrusted civil rights or privileges (Birmingham, 1840: 6).

The link was made even stronger when O'Connell himself on October 1840 took the pledge (Malcolm, 1986: 129; Quinn, 1992: 548), but began to weaken in 1843 when he said he needed to break the pledge, on doctor's orders (Malcolm, 1986: 130; Quinn, 1992: 548). At this stage, O'Connell began publicly to criticise the movement for its over-emphasis on the Irish being a 'drunken people' whereas in fact 'parliamentary figures' showed that 'the Scots drank considerably more' (Malcolm, 1986: 130).

O'Connell may have been critical of the movement, but 'he was careful not to criticise Father Mathew personally' (Malcolm, 1986: 130), perhaps because of Father Mathew's great popularity among the people. By contrast, the Catholic hierarchy were often at odds with Father Mathew, and purposely chose another candidate as bishop of Cork at a time when the local parish priests canvassed strongly on his behalf. Because of a lack of support from his superiors, the onslaught of the Great Famine, and other difficulties, Father Mathew's campaign was to deteriorate and die well before its charismatic advocate passed away himself (Father Mathew passed away in 1856).[5]

Drunkenness, the 'enemy of the human race', had been identified and needed to be erased (Birmingham, 1840: 54). Moreover, the drunkard was increasingly considered insane, rather than criminal, and, 'with the establishment of a national system of mental hospitals throughout Ireland during the nineteenth century from 1830 to the 1880s', the 'lunatic poor' found themselves in mental asylums, rather than 'poorhouses or prisons' (Walsh, 1989: 398). As Walsh points out '[a] survey of the hospital registers at the time shows that "intemperance and whiskey" were frequently given as supposed causes of patients' insanity' (1989: 398). The cure for insanity, physicians believed, was the asylum.

> They would teach discipline, a sense of limits and a satisfaction with one's position. . . The psychiatrists . . . conceived of proper individual behavior and social relationships only in terms of a personal respect for authority and tradition and an acceptance of one's station in the ranks of society. In this sense they were trying to re-create in the asylum their own vision of the colonial community. The results, however, were very different. Regimentation, punctuality, and precision became the asylum's basic traits, and these qualities were far more in keeping with an urban, industrial order than a local agrarian one. (Rothman, 1971: 154)

Throughout this time there were increasing calls for asylums specifically for inebriates. In Britain and Ireland, these notions of institutionalising inebriates gained popularity near the end of the nineteenth century, and culminated in the introduction of the Inebriates Act of 1898. This act 'consolidated earlier legislation and created a three-tiered system consisting of retreats meant for voluntary patients, and reformatories' (divided into two categories: certified reformatories and state institutions) 'intended for what might be called the "criminally drunk"' (Bretherton, 1986: 473). One year later, the State Inebriate Reformatory was established in Ennis.

Originally a county prison, the Ennis reformatory was converted under the General Prisons Board, 'administered as part of the system, and its officials and staff were drawn from that bureaucracy, a most telling fact, and a significant anomaly in the planning and operation of a scheme whose purpose was curative rather than punitive' (Bretherton, 1986: 483). The ideal for the institutional model was the hospital, where the 'staff might resemble turnkeys or warders in fact, but in theory they should look something more like orderlies or nurses' (Bretherton, 1986: 482). Traditionally in Ireland the Catholic Church assumed 'nursing, custodial or charity roles . . . and the certified inebriates' reformatories were another example of that role' (Smith, 1989: 58). Ennis had three chaplains: Catholic, Church of Ireland, and Presbyterian. The majority of the patients were women and were 'ministered to by the Sisters of Mercy, who were allowed to enter freely' (Smith, 1989: 61). In 1907 a Presbyterian chaplain had the following to say of the institution and its inmates:

There can be no doubt of the salutary influence of the Reformatory treatment upon those who are sent to it from time to time. The enforced absence from drink, the wholesome food, the simple life, the congenial employment, together with all the good influences exerted by the officials and chaplains – all these things make for the well-being of the inmates (Quoted in Bretherton, 1986: 484).

Two other reformatories opened in Ireland, largely, as Smith says, due to the involvement of the Catholic Church. However, like Ennis, these institutions were never used to their full capacity. In the years following the First World War, these institutions seemed to fade gradually on both sides of the Atlantic. Clearly in decline, the Ennis institution was transferred over to the military 'due to the exigencies of the Anglo-Irish War (1920)', and never reopened as an institution for the care of inebriates (Smith, 1989: 64).

The turning point for the treatment of individuals 'addicted' to 'intoxicants' in the Republic occurred with the enactment of the Mental Treatment Act of 1945 (Éire, 1945). Prior to this time, as Dr O'Higgins said during the Oireachtas debates surrounding this bill, 'those suffering from mental disease, if not definitely labelled as criminals, were treated somewhat worse than criminals, and our mental hospitals, or lunatic asylums as they were called at the time, were not treatment centres. They were places of detention.' (29 November, 1944: 1134). ' "[I]ntemperance and whiskey" were frequently given as supposed causes of patients' insanity', as Walsh observed in a survey of nineteenth-century hospital registers (1989: 398). Walsh goes on to say 'the Mental Treatment Act of 1945 gave formal recognition to alcoholism as a specific disorder requiring treatment and acknowledged that it was sometimes a characteristic of this disorder that the patient did not realise that he was ill and needed treatment providing for the compulsory admission and detention of alcoholics in mental hospitals as addicts' (1989: 398). An addict is defined in the act as a person who

(*a*) by reason of his addiction to drugs or intoxicants is either dangerous to himself or others or incapable of managing himself or his affairs or of ordinary proper conduct, or

(*b*) by reason of his addiction to drugs, intoxicants or perverted conduct is in serious danger of mental disorder.

The terminology is specifically vague to cover all forms of 'addiction', including 'alcohol addiction' or 'alcoholism'. In fact, the terms alcoholic or alcoholism never appear in the act; alcohol was not even an important issue in the government debates preceding the introduction of the Act. However, it should be noted that this act was touted, in the words of Dr Ward (the main author and government representative in charge of the bill), as 'the most advanced and, though I say it, the most enlightened code in any country in Europe' (Dáil Éireann Debate, 1945: 1398). This point indicates that they had looked extensively at the issue, and its treatment in other countries. In fact, there is a point to be made that the preferred term at the time was 'alcohol addiction' (Bales, 1980[1944]). Although the term 'alcoholism' had been around since the nineteenth century, it is reasonable to suggest that the widespread current day usage of the term is largely attributed to the promotion put forth by Alcoholics Anonymous.

AA and Drinking in Modern Ireland

The very next year AA was to arrive in Ireland. AA was founded in America in 1935 by Bill (William G. Wilson) and Dr Bob (Robert L. Smith, MD), both of whom considered themselves to be 'hopeless drunks' and believed that drunks could help other drunks to achieve sobriety through 'developing a supportive, open, frank, and spiritual fellowship committed primarily to that end' (Conrad and Schneider, 1980: 88).[6] The organisation expanded greatly, particularly after the publication of Bill's, Dr Bob's, and 27 other individuals' 'recovery stories' (Maxwell, 1982; Alcoholics Anonymous, 1939). The organisation was given further legitimation by its association with the Yale School for Alcohol Studies. Bill was invited to give a talk in 1944 at the first summer school for alcohol studies, at which time it was estimated that membership was 'approaching 15,000, with groups in over 360 places, including some in Canada' (Maxwell, 1982: 295). In the year that followed it was to spread to Australia, which directly contributed to its establishment in Ireland, the first European AA group.

While home visiting, Father Tom Dunlea (an Irish parish priest based in Australia), gave an interview to the Dublin paper, the *Evening Mail* (5 October, 1946), in which he discussed how he had been impressed with the success of AA in Sydney (Alcoholics Anonymous of Ireland, 1992: 5). After reading this interview, Conor F., an Irish immigrant member of AA in the United States back home for the holidays, decided before he returned to America that he was going to start an AA group in Dublin. Eventually Conor was directed to Dr Norman Moore, the head of St Patrick's Hospital in Dublin, who had read about AA in *Readers Digest* (Alcoholics Anonymous of Ireland, 1992: 6). Dr Moore introduced Conor to one of his patients, Richard P., and 'the two men "clicked" ' (Alcoholics Anonymous of Ireland, 1992: 6).

> They collected four or five men, started meeting in the home of one of them and eventually held the first Irish AA public meeting. About 45 people attended and at the end of it, some 12 'joined' up (Alcoholics Anonymous of Ireland, 1992: 6).

This first meeting was on 25 November 1946. After the holiday season, Conor F. returned to the United States, and the group was left to fend for themselves.

After this initial meeting, membership declined for the first eight months, at which point the group increased its level of advertising. By 1950, it was reported that there were twelve groups throughout Ireland, with approximately 1000 members (Alcoholics Anonymous of Ireland, 1996). Today it is estimated that there are approximately 700 groups across Ireland, with an estimated membership of 11,000 (personal communication with Alcoholics Anonymous of Ireland, 1996). Membership has continuously grown over the last fifty years, particularly in the 1960s and the 1970s, which, as I will discuss later, is the time period when alcohol consumption and hospitalisation rates also began to rise in Ireland.

The early academic study of alcoholism within Ireland is tied to AA. One of the first modern articles to be published on alcoholism in Ireland was written by Perceval (1955) who was described as an 'Honorary Social Psychiatric Worker, St Patrick's Hospital, Dublin', and was in fact the original Richard P., although his connection is not revealed in his article. There are numerous interesting and useful points made in this article about drinking and alcoholism, which he says was beginning at the time 'to be regarded as an illness rather than a moral defect' due to the publicity generated by AA (Perceval, 1955: 150). In fact, he points to AA as being the main treatment available to the alcoholics unable to pay for private treatment, although he does point out that there was an 'increased interest on the part of the younger general practitioners in the diagnosis and treatment of the disease of alcoholism' which was resulting in increased hospitalisation rates. These increased rates were used as evidence of 'the fact' that alcoholism was a 'serious national social problem' both by Perceval and by some of his successors, such as Walsh (1968; 1969).

Research on alcoholism in Ireland was basically non-existent until the latter part of the 1960s, and was in many ways connected to the establishment of both the *Medico-Social Research Board*[7] and *The Economic and Social Research Institute* (ESRI)[8] in Dublin. An early member of the *Medico-Social Research Board* was Dermot Walsh, who conducted an analysis of hospitalisation rates both in Dublin (1968) and in Ireland in general (1969). Specifically Walsh analysed the first admissions for alcoholism in Ireland for the year 1964, which he concluded were much higher than comparative figures for Scotland, or England and Wales. Although formal statistics are not available before 1965, we can see that, after that year and until recently, there was a continual rise in the admissions for both men and women. As Figure 1 shows, this rate seems to have peaked in 1984, and has been dropping ever since.

Looking through the annual reports of psychiatric hospitals, we see that between 1965 and 1970, alcoholic disorders were the fourth most popular diagnosis, behind Schizophrenia, Manic Depressive and Neurosis. In 1971 alcoholic disorders moved up to third position, passing out Neurosis, until 1975 when it moved up to second most popular, only behind Schizophrenia. Two years later, alcoholic disorders became the most popular diagnosis, a position it continued to hold until 1982 when Manic Depressive became the

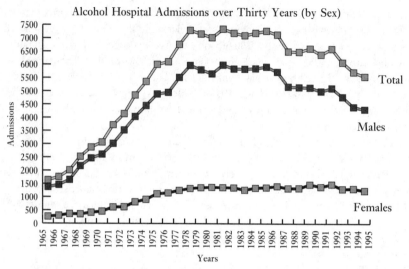

Figure 1: *Health Research Board's Annual Reports of Irish Psychiatric Hospitals and Units for various years.*

most popular diagnosis, followed by alcoholic disorders. Briefly in 1989 these two disorders switched places, but the following year, alcoholic disorders were again behind Manic Depressive. In 1994, the most recent available figures indicate that alcoholic disorders are now third most popular, behind Manic Depressive and Schizophrenia.

A gender breakdown of the diagnoses to psychiatric hospitals over the last three decades reveals that for males, alcoholic disorders moved to the second most popular diagnosis in 1967, behind only Schizophrenia. Five years later alcoholic disorders were to become the most popular diagnosis for Irish males and it has remained so ever since. For Irish women, alcoholic disorders moved up to fourth most popular diagnosis in 1973, behind Manic Depressive, Schizophrenia and Neurosis. This continued until 1986 when alcoholic disorders moved up to be third most popular diagnosis, displacing Neurosis. However, in 1993, alcoholic disorders were to move back down to fourth most popular, behind Manic Depressive, Schizophrenia and Mania. These statistics seem to indicate a double gender bias. Women are more likely to be diagnosed with some form of depressive disorder, while males seem to be more readily diagnosed with some form of alcoholic disorder.

Generally, in Irish society there seems to be less social stigma attached to alcohol-related problems than general psychiatric diagnosis, particularly for males. Recently, Saris (1995) talked about the hierarchical structure of patients in psychiatric institutions in Ireland – within this group, alcoholics are considered to have the highest status, and schizophrenics the lowest. Similarly, one psychiatric nurse told me that 'everyone in for alcohol problems has something else wrong with them'. Recently, Dermot Walsh, the Department of Health's inspector of mental hospitals, said that 'drink problems which were seen by various agencies – families, guards, employers – to be difficult and a nuisance were just clapped off into psychiatric hospitals', and that people with alcohol-related problems should be treated elsewhere (Kerr, 1994: A9).[9]

Probably the first study to specifically challenge the notion of widespread alcoholism among the Irish was Lynn and Hampson's (1970) article. Although they acknowledge that Dublin's psychiatric admissions for alcoholism were higher than England and Wales and Scotland, they said that they were lower than Helsinki and Canada. Furthermore, Lynn and Hampson presented data showing that, in comparison to many other countries, Ireland had low rates for deaths from alcoholism and cirrhosis of the liver, convictions for drunkenness, and per capita consumption. In conclusion they said that all these statistics indicated lack of support 'for the common assumption that alcohol consumption and alcoholism are exceptionally prevalent in Ireland' (1970: 392). In fact, at that time, the per capita consumption figures had recently been considered by American researchers to be specifically related to national rates of alcoholism.

The work of a French statistician, Ledermann (1956; 1964; 1965), had recently become known to the English-speaking world, and in turn was sending shock waves, still being felt throughout the field of alcohol studies. Ledermann argued that there was a direct and simple relationship between national rates of cirrhosis of the liver and overall national consumption statistics. Specifically he advocated that the lowering of the latter would reduce the former. In his original work, published only in French, he clearly showed that there was a direct cross-cultural statistical link between cirrhosis of the liver rates and alcohol deaths. Less convincingly, Ledermann also tried to show a relationship between mortality rates for cirrhosis of the liver and consumption rates. However, he committed a commonly recognised error of data collected over time: he drew causal inferences from a time-series relationship between two variables that have a consistent trend over time, ignoring the possibility of external factors that may be influencing both of them.

Perhaps the main point that Ledermann made, though, was that the distribution of the amount of drinking in any population follows a single log-normal curve, and that average consumption and heavy consumption covary. Thus, Ledermann argued, there was a simple mathematical relationship between the proportion of heavy drinkers and the average consumption of a given population.

There are, however, serious problems with the formulas which Ledermann offered due to the fact that he did not take into account the standard deviation within the population. One researcher summed this up by saying that 'neither the dispersion nor the number of heavy consumers of a population can be uniquely determined by the mean consumption' (Skog, 1977: 11). Another researcher argued, along the same lines, that per capita measures of consumption must be related to societal drinking patterns, and should take into account variables such as age and sex distributions in the populations (Pittman, 1980). The model has been criticised as well on the basis of the reliability of consumption rates cross-culturally, especially since they do not take into account illegal or legal home production of alcoholic beverages (Pittman, 1980). Pittman (1987) has also raised the question of policies directed towards reducing the consumption of drinkers 'who experience no negative consequences' from their drinking. Gusfield has even equated the emergence of this perspective as the 'new temperance movement' due to its emphasis on 'raising control measures, including availability of alcoholic beverages' (1984: 411). These notions were, and to some degree still are, attractive to some government agencies and policy-makers.

Ireland still has a comparatively low per capita consumption rate, although it has been rising over the last thirty years and, as Table 1 shows, has by far the lowest cirrhosis of the liver mortality rates for either males or females.

Table 1: *Sex Difference in Rates of Mortality due to Chronic Liver Diseases and Cirrhosis (per 100,000 population)*

Country	Males	Females	Year
Ireland	3.5	1.8	(1992)
Northern Ireland*	5.0	3.7	(1992)
England and Wales	7.0	5.0	(1992)
Scotland	10.2	7.3	(1992)
Denmark**	18.4	9.7	(1993)
Finland	14.9	6.0	(1993)
France	22.7	9.7	(1992)
Germany	32.6	16.2	(1992)
Greece	14.6	6.5	(1992)
Italy	34.4	19.2	(1991)
Netherlands	6.3	4.0	(1992)
Norway	6.0	3.6	(1992)
Poland	15.9	7.3	(1993)
Portugal	41.8	14.7	(1993)
Spain	28.2	11.8	(1991)
Sweden	9.5	4.3	(1991)

Note: *Northern Ireland figures are based on unadjusted population figures.
          **Danish rates are for Cirrhosis of Liver only.
Source: World Health Organization, 1995; except Northern Ireland, England and Wales, and Scotland figures which came from the Office of Population Censuses and Surveys, 1994.

These low figures have always existed in Ireland. In fact, another early study to come out of the *Medico-Social Research Boards* was done by Duffy and Dean; specifically set out to address the issue of the reliability of mortality statistics in Ireland and the possibility 'that low mortality from cirrhosis could be due to inaccurate reporting of the cause of death on the death certificate' (1971: 393). They concluded that Irish death certificates were not biased in their representation of cirrhosis, and said that by any 'international standard Ireland has a low mortality from cirrhosis of the liver' (1971: 396).

Moderation and Policy

In an interview given to the *British Journal of Addiction* in the mid-1980s, Mark Keller, an early and influential member of the Yale school, had the following to say when asked 'What have been the real underlying changes in society's attitudes to drinking and drinking problems?'

> There are fashions in the way of looking at things. We had a time when alcohol was blamed for everything. It was blamed for poverty, it was blamed for crime, it was blamed for disease, and this led to doing something extreme and eventually to Prohibition. That produced such problems that you had to get rid of Prohibition. And there followed a reversal of viewpoint. There followed a period when alcohol was unblamed by everyone – it's not alcohol which is causing diseases, it's the lack of vitamins. It's not alcohol which is causing the poverty, it's that the poverty is causing people to drink, and so on. I think that actually we are now beginning to see the next reversal, so alcohol is again beginning to be blamed for everything. Therefore I think I can predict that after a period of time we will have another shift to unblaming (Keller, 1985: 8–9).

The current move towards sensible or moderate drinking, I believe, is the shift to unblaming that Keller predicted.

Connected with these ideas has been a growing public health message, in Europe particularly, of the advocation of 'sensible drinking'. In 1994, these issues were debated in the World Health Forum, and the organising discussion was given by the Irish researcher Joyce O'Connor. First, O'Connor argued the need to develop a 'healthy public policy' related to alcohol that would involve 'the dissemination of information related to drinking' (1994: 214). Further, she said it would be necessary to create 'a climate where sensible drinking is the norm and is seen as the appropriate type of behaviour' (O'Connor, 1994: 215). These changes would necessitate the education of individuals regarding behaviours they may take for granted. Finally, O'Connor argued that both communities and health services need to be involved in this entire process.

Recently the Irish government released a long anticipated *National Alcohol Policy* (September, 1996). Based on information and guidelines in keeping with the World Health Organisation's research and the European Charter on Alcohol, the policy is specifically 'directed at reducing the prevalence of alcohol-related problems and thereby promoting the health of the community' (Department of Health, 1996: 59).

> The aim is to influence people's attitudes and habits so that, for those who choose to drink, moderate drinking becomes personally and socially acceptable and favoured in the Irish culture. Measures targeting the whole population as well as specific at risk groups are required. No single measure will be effective if taken in isolation. High prices and restriction on the availability of alcohol are the most effective measures but cannot be sustained long term without public support through information and advocacy. Measures targeting specific groups, especially young people, and specific settings such as [the] workplace, along with accessible and effective treatment services ensure a comprehensive policy (Department of Health, 1996: 59).

In keeping with recommendations of a 1984 report on psychiatric services, the report recommends the establishment of community-based services, encouraging health boards to:

- Establish at least one alcohol/drug resource centre in each community care area.
- Give responsibility to a designated consultant psychiatrist with a special interest in alcohol.
- Provide a comprehensive therapy to the client and his/her family and friends, together with an after-care service.
- Ensure, wherever possible, that detoxification take place on an outpatient basis.

                              (Department of Health, 1996: 65).

The report also makes the important point that '[t]here is no one treatment that is clearly more effective than any other' (Department of Health, 1996: 38). Research does not definitely show a significant difference between the various treatment models. In fact, the most recent research advocates flexibility on the part of the health-care provider with a view to matching clients to treatments (Linstrm, 1992).

Notes

1 In comparison, the term alcohol dates back to the sixteenth century, and originally referred to 'the fine metallic powder used in the East to stain the eyelids' (OED, 1933: 209). By extension the term in early Chemistry began to be used to refer to 'any fine impalpable powder produced by trituration or especially by sublimation'. Thus the term was extended to refer to fluids that had undergone 'distillation or "rectification"'; such fluids, also brought from the East, appear to have arrived around the same time in Europe.

2 The term 'alcoholic' appeared in 1790, more than a century after the term 'alcohol' had been introduced, but seems to have been originally used mainly in chemistry to mean 'of or belonging to alcohol' (OED, 1933: 210). Its use to refer to 'one afflicted with alcoholism' does not come into use until the 1890s (Merriam-Webster, 1989: 69).

3 I have argued elsewhere (Cassidy, 1997) that the ambiguity of the concept 'alcoholism', and the underlying medical notions of 'the disease model', allowed an eventual unity between the disparate moral stands surrounding alcohol issues. On the one side, the temperance/medical body, particularly in America, originally saw a need for social controls of the product, but in other countries and after Prohibition in America, their efforts were directed towards the drinker. At the other end of the moral spectrum were researchers who saw the long-standing and deep-rooted ritualistic and symbolic meanings associated with the majority of uses of alcohol in most drinking nations. These positive social uses became the staple images of the drinks industry, and of the commercial drinking body which was formed at the same time that the temperance/medical body was emerging (Lyon and Barbalet, 1994).

4 In Rush's famous work *Inquiry into the Effects of Ardent Spirits* (1790), he gave a 'moral and physical thermometer' of various alcoholic beverages. The safest things to consume which lead to 'temperance, health and wealth' were water, followed by milk, small beer (this refers to weak beer), cider, wine, porter and strong beer. Those beverages which lead to intemperance, vices, diseases, and punishments were punch, toddy and egg rum, grog (brandy and water), gin, brandy and rum.

5 Father Mathew's name was resurrected in 1898 by Father James Cullen who established the Pioneers Total Abstinence Association. This association has continued to have a large influence on Irish society, with approximately a quarter to a third of the population totally abstaining from alcohol. Pioneers say a daily prayer for the sins of the intemperate, although they fully condone the moderate use of alcohol. Pioneers maintain loose associations with organisations specifically for alcoholics, such as AA, and alcoholics who have abstained from alcohol for a suitable period of time are eligible for membership. Beyond spiritual help, Pioneers do not see themselves as having a role in reaching this sobriety.

6 Anonymity is a principle associated with Bill's original vision of the organisation, and is associated with the stigma which was originally attached to the issue.

7 This group began in 1966. In 1986 the *Medico-Social Research Board* and the *Medical Research Council of Ireland* merged to form the *Health Research Board* (personal communication with the Health Research Board, Dublin).

8 The ESRI began in 1960 (Kennedy, 1985).

9 'Guards', as used here, is a colloquial Anglicisation of 'Gardai'. The Gardai, or Gardai Siochana, are the Irish police force.

References

Anonymous (1939) *Alcoholics Anonymous.* New York: Works Publishing Company.

Alcoholics Anonymous of Ireland (1992) *AA Service Manual.* Dublin: The General Service Board of Alcoholics Anonymous of Ireland.

Bales, Robert F. (1946) Cultural difference in rates of alcoholism, *Quarterly Journal of Studies on Alcohol,* 6: 480–99.

Bales, Robert F. (1962) Attitudes towards drinking in Irish culture, in: David J. Pittman, and Charles R. Snyder (eds) *Society, Culture and Drinking Patterns.* New York: John Wiley.

Bales, Robert F. (1980[1944]) *The 'Fixation Factor' in Alcohol Addiction: An Hypothesis Derived from a Comparative Study of Irish and Jewish Social Norms,.* New York: Arno Press.

Birmingham, James (1840) *A Memoir of the Very Rev. Theobald Mathew,* Dublin: Milliken.

Blaney, Roger (1973–74) Alcoholism in Ireland: medical and social aspects, *Journal of the Statistical and Social Inquiry Society of Ireland,* 23: 108–24.

Bretherton, George Cornell (1986) Irish inebriate reformatories, 1899–1920: a small experiment in coercion, *Contemporary Drug Problems,* 13: 473–502.

Bretherton, George Cornell (1991) Against the flowing tide: whiskey and temperance in making modern Ireland, in: Susanna Barrows and Room Robin (eds) *Drinking: Behaviour and Belief in Modern History.* Berkeley: University of California Press.

Cassidy, Tanya M. (1996) Irish drinking worlds: a socio-cultural reinterpretation of ambivalence, *International Journal of Sociology and Social Policy,* 16(5/6): 5–25.

Cassidy, Tanya M. (1997) 'Alcohol in Ireland. The Irish Solution', Unpublished PhD thesis, University of Chicago.

Conniffe, Denis and Daniel McCoy (1993) *Alcohol Use in Ireland: Some Economic and Social Implications.* General Research Series Paper No. 160, Dublin: Economic and Social Research Institute.

Conrad, Peter and Joseph W. Schneider (1980) *Deviance and Medicalization: From Badness to Sickness,* St Louis: C.V. Mosby.

Dáil Éireann (1944) *Díospóireacta Pálaiminte (Parliamentary Debates),* Dublin: Tuairisc Oifigiil (Official Report), 95, 29 November: 1079–1135.

Department of Health (1996) *National Alcohol Policy,* Dublin: Stationery Office.

Duffy, George J. and Geoffrey Dean (1971) The reliability of death certification of cirrhosis, *Journal of the Irish Medical Association.* 64 (417): 393–7.

Éire (1945) Mental Treatment Act, 1945, in: *The Acts of the Oireachtas Passed in the Year 1945,* Number 19 of 1945, Dublin: Stationery Office.

Foucault, Michel (1967) *Madness and Civilisation: A History of Madness in the Age of Reason.* London: Tavistock.

Foucault, Michel (1977) *Discipline and Punish: The Birth of the Prison.* London: Tavistock.

Gronbaek M, A. Deis, T.I.A. Sorensen, U. Becker, K.B. Johnsen, C. Muller, *et al.* (1994) Influence of sex, age, body mass index, and smoking on alcohol intake and mortality, *British Medical Journal,* 308: 302–6.

Gusfield, Joseph (1984) Prevention: rise, decline and renaissance, in: E.L.Gomberg, H.R. White and J.A. Carpenter (eds) *Alcohol, Science and Society Revisited.* Ann Arbor: University of Michigan Press.

Keller, Mark (1982) On defining alcoholism: with comment on some other relevant words, in: E.L.Gomberg, H.R.White and J.A. Carpenter (eds) *Alcohol, Science and Society Revisited.* Ann Arbor: University of Michigan Press.

Keller, Mark (1985) Journal interview, 8: Conversation with Mark Keller, *British Journal of Addiction*, 80: 5–9.

Keller, Mark and Mairi McCormick (1968) *A Dictionary of Words about Alcohol*. New Brunswick: Rutgers Center of Alcohol Studies.

Kennedy, Kieran A. (1985) Twenty-five years of economic and social research, *Bulletin of the Department of Foreign Affairs*, Dublin: Economic and Social Research Institute.

Kerr, Colin (1994) Mental units 'misused': treat drinkers elsewhere says doctor. *The Sunday Tribune*, 30 January.

Kerrigan, Colm (1992) *Father Mathew and the Irish Temperance Movement 1838–1849*. Cork: Cork University Press.

Ledermann, Sully (1956) *Alcohol, Alcoolisme, Alcoolisation. Vol.1. Données scientifiques de caractère physiologiques économique et social* [Alcohol, Alcoholism, Alcoholization. Vol.1. Scientific Data of the Physiological, Economic, and Social Character], Institut National d'Etudes Démographiques; Travauz et Documents, Cahier no. 29, Paris: Presses Universitaires de France.

Ledermann, Sully (1964) *Alcohol, Alcoolisme, Alcoolisation. Vol.2. Mortalité, morbidité, accidents du Travail* [Alcohol, Alcoholism, Alcoholization. Vol.2. Mortality, Morbitity, and Work Related Accidents], Institut National d'Etudes Démographiques; Travauz et Documents, Cahier no.41, Paris: Presses Universitaires de France.

Ledermann, Sully (1965) Can one reduce alcoholism without changing total alcohol consumption in a population? in: *Selected Papers Presented at the 27th International Congress on Alcohol and Alcoholism, Frankfurt 1964*. Vol.2, Lausanne: International Council on Alcohol and Alcoholism.

Levine, Harry Gene (1978) The discovery of addiction: changing conceptions of habitual drunkenness in America, *Journal of Studies on Alcohol*, 39(1): 143–74.

Linström, Lars (1992) *Managing Alcoholism: Matching Clients to Treatments*. Oxford: Oxford University Press.

Lyon, M.L. and J.M. Barbalet (1994) Society's body: emotion and the 'somatization' of social theory, in: Thomas J.Csordas (ed.) *Embodiment and Experience: The Existential Ground of Culture and Self*. Cambridge: Cambridge University Press.

Lynn, R. and S. Hampson (1970) Alcoholism and alcohol consumption in Ireland, *Journal of the Irish Medical Association*, 63(392): 39–42.

Maguire, John Francis (1863) *Father Mathew: A Biography*. London: Longmann, Roberts, and Green.

Malcolm, Elizabeth (1986) *'Ireland Sober, Ireland Free': Drink and Temperance in Nineteenth-Century Ireland*. Dublin: Gill & Macmillan.

Maxwell, Milton A. (1982) Alcoholics anonymous, in: E.L.Gomberg, H.R. White and J.A. Carpenter (eds) *Alcohol, Science and Society Revisited*. Ann Arbor: University of Michigan Press.

Merriam-Webster (1989) *Webster's Ninth New Collegiate Dictionary*, Springfield Mass: Merriam-Webster.

O'Connor, Joyce (1994) Sensible drinking. *World Health Forum* Volume 15, 213–32.

Oxford English Dictionary (OED) (1933) Oxford: Clarendon Press.

Pittman, D. (1967) International overview: social and cultural factors in drinking patterns, pathological and nonpathological, in: D. Pittman (ed.) *Alcoholism*. New York: Harper and Row.

Pittman, D. (1980) *Primary Prevention of Alcohol Abuse and Alcoholism: An Evaluation of the Control of Consumption Policy*. St Louis: Washington University Social Science Institute.

Pittman, D.(1987) Sensible alcohol policy, *British Journal of Addiction*, 82: 1289–91.

Plant, M. (1990) *Women and Alcohol – A Review of International Literature on the Use of Alcohol by Females*, WHO Regional Office for Europe, EUR/ICP.ADA 020.

Quinn, John F.(1992) The 'vagabond friar': Father Mathew's difficulties with the Irish bishops, 1840–1856, *The Catholic Historical Review*, 78: 542–56.

Renaud, Serge and Michel de Lorgeril (1992) Wine, alcohol, platelets and the French paradox for coronary heart disease, *Lancet*, 339: 1523–6.

Rothman, D.J. (1971) *The Discovery of the Asylum*. Boston: Little, Brown and Co.

Rush, Benjamin (1943[1785]) An inquiry into the effects of ardent spirits upon the human body and mind, *Quarterly Journal of Studies on Alcohol*, 4: 321–41.

Saris, A. Jamie (1995) Telling stories: life histories, illness narratives, and institutional landscapes. *Culture, Medicine and Psychiatry*, 19(1): 39–72.

Single, Eric (1995) Harm reduction and alcohol, *International Journal of Drug Policy*, 6(1):1–5.

Skog, O.-J.(1977) On the distribution of alcohol consumption, *National Institute for Alcohol Research*, No.4, Oslo.

Smith, B.A. (1989) Ireland's Ennis inebriates' reformatory: A 19th century example of failed institutional reform, *Federal Probation*. 53(1): 53–64.

Trotter, T. (1941[1804]) Classics of the alcohol literature. An early medical view of alcohol addiction and its treatment. Dr Thomas Trotter's 'Essay, medical, philo-sophical and chemical, on drunkenness', *Quarterly Journal of Studies on Alcohol*, 2: 584–91.

Walsh, Dermot (1969) Alcoholism in the Republic of Ireland, *The British Journal of Psychiatry*, 115(526):1021–5.

Walsh, Dermot (1989) Alcoholism and the Irish, in: Mac Marshall (ed.) *Beliefs, Behaviors and Alcoholic Beverages: A Cross-cultural Survey*. Ann Arbor: University of Michigan Press.

12

Gender differences in Mental Health in Ireland

Anne Cleary

Introduction

Durkheim's (1951) study of suicide, published in 1897, marked the beginning of sociological research in the area of mental health. Durkheim focused on suicide to give credentials to the new discipline of sociology and demonstrated how sociological factors could explain patterns in suicide rates within and between countries. This tradition – the study of trends in mental disorder – continued in the twentieth century in the social-epidemiological work of Faris and Dunham (1939) and later Hollingshead and Redlich (1958). Although this social causation approach to the study of health and illness remains a significant aspect of sociological inquiry, other approaches are now equally important. From the mid-twentieth century, sociologists turned their attention to a much wider landscape which involved examining the socially constructed nature of health and disease and this necessitated a move away from medical definitions of disorder. In this way labelling theorists such as Goffman (1961) offered an account of madness from the point of view of the 'disordered' and Michel Foucault's (1967) work further deconstructed the concepts of illness and disorder linking them to the development and maintenance of medical discourse and power. This overall shift in perspective has been viewed as a move from the study of sociology-*in*-medicine to the sociology *of* medicine and is now usually referred to as the Sociology of Health and Illness.

The labelling perspective provided the first strand in the development of sociological interest in gender and mental disorder. Another line of inquiry emerged from within feminist writing. Initial feminist interest centred on the apparent over-representation of women in mental health statistics and the links between this and patriarchal features in society. This framework has developed in a number of ways but an important aspect is the notion that mental disorder is a distinctively feminine condition. This concept of the 'feminisation of madness' can be seen in various evolutionary stages in the work of Chesler (1972) , Showalter (1987) and Ussher (1991). Showalter's (1987) work in particular has received a good deal of attention because of her claim, based on the over representation of women in nineteenth- and twentieth-century (English) hospital statistics, that this 'feminisation of madness' originated in the nineteenth century. Feminist analysis has continued to focus on female aspects of mental disorder while male dimensions have, in general, received much less attention. In fact the prominence of studies of female mental disorder in recent years has resulted in a situation in which male mental disorder sometimes appears to be insignificant by comparison. There are of course important exceptions to this and some writers have considered both male and female mental disorder (Smith, 1975; Busfield, 1996). Recent developments in sociology – particularly the sociology of gender – have prompted further interest in both male and female manifestations of distress and disorder.

The background summary illustrates the various themes involved in this area of inquiry but also points to the problematic nature of the topic. Firstly, competing paradigms operate, and data can, and have, been used or emphasised to prove various theories (Smith, 1975). Much theoretical work has developed from the apparent finding that women generally outnumber men in mental health statistics. The origins of this theory may be traced to the work of Gove and Tudor (1973) and also Chesler (1972) in the 1970s. Both presented data which purported to show that more women than men were affected by (or labelled as) mentally disordered. However these findings were soon contested by Smith (1975) and others (Dohrenwend and Dohrenwend, 1976) who noted that the female excess was restricted to certain diagnostic categories of mental disorder, in particular depression and neurosis. This conclusion remains a consistent research finding (Kessler *et al.*,1993; Weissman *et al.*, 1993). Nevertheless, even this over-representation has been challenged. Firstly, cross-cultural studies have not been extensive and some research has produced contrasting findings, with higher male rates of disorder (Orley and Wing, 1979; Weissman and Klerman, 1977). Secondly, even within similar cultures not all studies show the same pattern. American research indicates that the over-representation of women in depression is not true of black women or other racial groups (Comstock and Helsing 1978, Linn *et al.*,1979, Dressler and Badger 1985) or of particular subcultures (Egeland and Hostetter, 1983). Thirdly, some researchers (from the UK and elsewhere) dispute a genuine female excess in this category of disorder (Parker, 1979: Jenkins, 1985). They claim instead that much of the excess is due to the fact that a wide spectrum of depressed mood states is included in the research definition of depression and any difference can be explained by variations in the way mental disorder is measured (Craig and Van Natta, 1979; Clark *et al.*, 1981). It is claimed that minor mood changes are more readily reported by women and this is seen, for instance, in studies which use instruments that depend on self-reported symptoms (rather than assessment by a psychiatrist) and which usually show higher female rates (Newmann, 1984). However, if the diagnostic evaluation is restricted to depression of clinical severity, the male-female disparity becomes considerably less (Jenkins, 1985).

The above discussion suggests a number of important points. Firstly, it is unlikely that female rates of mental disorder exceed male rates in general. Secondly, methodological and conceptual considerations are crucial in interpreting even diagnosis-specific data. The apparent excess of female rates is seen only in some populations and here different methodologies may have contributed to the seemingly discrepant findings. Hence, the statistical basis of any particular study is itself an important consideration. Findings based on hospital in-patient figures are particularly suspect as such figures merely denote those within the hospital system and are therefore a poor indicator of true prevalence. Data from 'community studies' are potentially more accurate but such figures are also dependent on the measuring instrument involved. In addition, community studies are also affected by 'illness behaviour' and by service provision factors. Finally, findings from studies may be interpreted differently. For instance, if women present in greater numbers for a particular condition, what exactly does this mean? It may simply indicate that men and women experience psychological difficulties in different ways. Here labelling and feminist theorists would be concerned with the categories or labels as well as with who is doing the labelling. Thus, it is claimed, more women are labelled mad either because of a general societal desire to regulate women or because of more localised sexist practices by medical practitioners (Chesler, 1972). Within the discourse of medicine, therefore, a male ideal of health exists and women are more likely to be categorised as 'unhealthy' or disordered (Penfold and Walker, 1984; Ehrenreich and English 1976).

Mental Disorder in Ireland

In Ireland we have a distinctive history of attitudes to and care of the mentally ill and this includes a particular gender dimension in relation to mental disorder. Ireland, in line with other European countries, adopted large scale hospitalisation of the mentally ill from the nineteenth century onwards but it may be said that we used this system somewhat more enthusiastically than other countries and maintained the system longer (Robins, 1986). The reasons for this are complex and discussed elsewhere in this book (Saris, pp. 208–23 below) but have had important implications for the study of mental disorder as available data are almost entirely confined to in-patient figures. One consequence of this has been an assumed higher incidence of schizophrenia in Ireland which has since been shown to be inaccurate. The higher rate of schizophrenia found in this country was due to the Irish tendency to hospitalise those with the condition (Ní Nualláin, *et al.* 1984). As the asylum system developed in Ireland during the nineteenth century there was a dramatic increase in in-patient numbers and more men than women were consistently admitted (Finnane, 1981). This pattern of (slightly) higher male admissions and residency was reflected in both the public (Finnane, 1981) and private asylum system (Malcolm, 1989). This is in contrast to the situation in England where hospital statistics in the nineteenth and twentieth centuries have shown a female preponderance (O'Hare and O'Connor, 1987; Busfield, 1996). In fact Showalter (1987) has used this female excess to map the origins of madness as a particularly female phenomenon. Any analysis based on in-patient figures is problematic. Nevertheless it is possible to discern in the Irish figures a gender pattern of male predominance based on admissions and residency and this has continued into the twentieth century (O'Hare and O'Connor, 1987). These trends therefore do not support Showalter's (1987) thesis that the regulation of women (rather than men) through the asylum system began in the nineteenth century.

If we try to draw a picture of the men and women who were hospitalised in the nineteenth century we have but a very hazy idea of their lives and experiences. Research work on the pattern of nineteenth-century hospitalisation (Finnane, 1981; Malcolm, 1989) has shown that those admitted were predominantly young and single, and, of those admitted to the public asylum system, mainly from the working or labouring classes (Finnane, 1981). There was a regional variation in admission rates, admissions being highest in Dublin and lowest in the west of Ireland. This pattern was reversed in the twentieth century with highest rates of admissions in the west of the country (O'Hare and O'Connor, 1987). There is some indication that by the end of the nineteenth century the asylum had begun to take on a regulatory role in Irish society. However, this appears to have applied not just to women but to men also. Violence or family conflict was a common precipitant of admission for men (Finnane, 1981) while for women, particularly single women, loss of financial support (due perhaps to the death of a father or husband) often preceded an admission (Malcolm, 1989). Ill health, including the health risks associated with pregnancy, was a frequent cause of admission for women and these admissions often had fatal consequences. In the nineteenth century, 6% of women died within the first three months of admission to the asylum, probably resulting from puerperal fever (Finnane, 1981). In summary then, by the beginning of the twentieth century the asylum had become an acknowledged part of Irish society and increasing rates of admissions, often resulting in long-term hospitalisation, set a trend of male predominance particularly in the west of Ireland (Finnane, 1981).

Table 1: *Gender and Diagnosis 1995. Admission rates per 100,000 population*.*

	Male	Female
Organic psychosis	24.4	22.2
Schizophrenia	193.7	123.0
Unspecified Psychoses	4.8	6.0
Depressive Disorders	169.4	246.1
Mania	67.6	83.4
Neurosis	38.0	51.5
Personality Disorders	39.6	39.6
Alcohol Disorders	222.3	77.0
Drug Dependence	23.1	7.5
Mental Handicap	26.5	11.6
Unspecified	10.8	12.7

* Source: Activities of Irish Psychiatric Hospitals and Units (Keogh and Walsh, 1996)

If recent Irish statistics in relation to psychiatric hospitals are examined, the general picture is one of a continued excess of male admissions (54%) (Keogh and Walsh, 1996). This male predominance extends to each health board area but is greatest along the western seaboard. However, a more gendered picture emerges if we explore the separate diagnostic categories detailed in Table 1. Here it can be seen that while more men are admitted for substance abuse (particularly alcoholism), more women are admitted for depression. These figures confirm findings from other studies (including the female/male rate for depression which approximates to the 2:1 ratio usually found) (Weissman *et al.*, 1993). Differences in relation to other categories including schizophrenia are smaller. The female/male differential for schizophrenia is somewhat greater than in England and elsewhere (Goldstein, 1992). Again, although personality disorder tends to be predominantly a male category elsewhere (Myers *et al.*,1984; Busfield, 1996), Irish figures do not support this. The two main diagnostic categories which show a definite gender patterning both in Ireland and elsewhere are therefore depressive disorders and substance abuse (alcoholism and drug dependence). These particular diagnostic categories are based to a considerable extent on evaluations of behaviour and therefore represent a more contested, and more flexible, area diagnostically. In addition, because they are often defined as 'problems in living' (Szasz, 1961) rather than psychiatric conditions, there is a possibility that gender considerations may influence the diagnosis (Broverman *et al.*, 1970).

By examining admissions to Irish psychiatric hospitals according to age and gender, it can be seen (Table 2) that the male predominance extends to nearly every age cohort. More males than females present for admission to psychiatric hospitals under the age of 15 years in both Ireland and England (DHSS, 1997). However, the female predominance in the older age categories in the UK is not

Table 2. *All Admissions, Age and Gender. Ireland 1995 (Per 100,000 population).**

	Male	Female
Under 15	52.6	16.4
15–19	252.6	184.0
20–24	790.6	565.7
25–34	1312.4	815.3
35–44	1423.6	1100.5
45–54	1474.0	1282.6
55–64	1269.9	1164.0
65–74	1077.7	1178.3
75 and over	866.5	996.6

*Source: Activities of Irish Psychiatric Hospitals and Units (Keogh and Walsh, 1995)

evident in Ireland. In the UK, more female admissions occur in each age category over 45 years (HMSO, 1997). A male predominance is also evident within Irish psychiatric hospitals if residency rates are considered (Moran and Walsh, 1992). The majority of psychiatric in-patients in Ireland are male (54.7%), outnumbering women in nearly all age cohorts except over 65 years, where the excess female rate reflects gender differences in mortality. Men are also more likely to become long-stay residents in that they comprise 56% of those who remain in hospital for more than one year. Although all psychiatric hospitals in Ireland have pursued a policy of de-institutionalisation there is evidence that men – particularly older men – do not easily forsake what they consider to be the security and regularity of hospital life (Cleary, 1987).

Additional evidence of gender differences comes from an examination of data from the Central Mental Hospital, Ireland's national forensic unit (Health Research Board, 1997). Data from this hospital show that males are over-whelmingly represented in this area of the psychiatric system. Although the number of males admitted has been falling during the 1990s, men still accounted for 84% of admissions to this sector in 1995 (from 91% in 1990) (Health Research Board, 1997). This channelling of men into the judicial psychiatric system is consistent with findings elsewhere. Men are much more likely to be channelled into this sector and women more likely to be directed away from this area of the psychiatric service (Allen, 1987). Conversely, if the private hospital system (Table 3) is highlighted, this area tends to be dominated by female admissions.

More women overall are admitted to private psychiatric hospitals (57% in contrast to 42% in health board hospitals) where female admission rates are higher than male rates in five of the ten diagnostic categories. In the remaining five categories, which include alcohol and drug abuse, male/female differences are quite small. The gender differential is greatest in two categories – depression

Table 3: *Admissions to Private Hospitals in Ireland 1995. Diagnosis and Gender.* *

	Total Admissions	% of Admissions	Females as % of Admissions
Organic psychosis	197	5	48
Schizophrenia	551	13	46
Unspecified Psychoses	19	0.5	79
Depressive Disorders	1275	30	69
Mania	520	12	59
Neurosis	377	9	66
Personality Disorders	137	0.3	69
Alcohol Abuse	876	21	41
Drug Dependence	77	9	43
Mental Handicap	33	0.8	42
Unspecified	182	4	63

*Source: Health Research Board, 1997.

and personality disorders. The figure for personality disorders is interesting as it indicates a different pattern to other sectors of the hospital system and to other countries (Busfield, 1996). However, in terms of overall numbers, depression is the most important category for female admissions. Depression is the most common admission category to Irish private hospitals comprising 30% of admissions (in contrast to 25% in health board hospitals). Over two thirds (69%) of these admissions are female. This finding prompts the question whether middle-class women (who are more likely to avail themselves of private hospital services) are more vulnerable to depression. Research evidence does not support this (Brown and Harris, 1978) and these figures may merely reflect differences in the types of service offered by the public and private hospital systems in Ireland. Alternatively, it could be argued that women who are admitted to the private hospital system suffer from a more severe form of depression but this, too, is unlikely. The more obvious conclusion is that these differences represent variations in treatment methods between the public and private sectors.

In summary, Irish hospital statistics do suggest a pattern influenced by gender. However, in-patient figures are insufficient to allow any definite conclusions and in order to pursue this examination of gender distribution more fully we must extend the analysis to the community.

Information relating to community incidence and prevalence is scarce in this country. The following figures are based on two case registers operated by the Health Research Board in Dublin and Roscommon which include both in-patient and out-patient presentations to the psychiatric services (O'Hare and O'Connor, 1987). In 1984 O'Hare and O'Connor (1987) analysed data from this source for the years 1974–82 and their paper raised interesting questions about the gender distribution of psychiatric morbidity. The main finding of their study was that the incidence of mental disorder including depression was higher for males than females in Roscommon while the reverse was true in Dublin. The authors suggested that the different rural pattern for depression might be due firstly to the traditional pattern of service presentation in the west of Ireland i.e. a higher than average number of male presentations generally. Secondly, they proposed that rural Irish women might have been using less stigmatising forms of help for psychological problems, that is, attending their general practitioner rather than a psychiatric out-patient clinic. However, the last year examined (1982) showed a small excess of women over men, and indicated a possible change in the previous pattern. The following table, which shows presentation rates into the 1990s (O'Hare and O'Connor, 1987; Health Research Board, 1997), provides evidence that this indeed was the beginning of a new trend.

Table 4. *Case Register Incidence, Roscommon and Dublin, for Depression by Gender 1974–1994 (Rates per 10,000 population over 15 years old)*.*

	Dublin		Roscommon	
	Female	Male	Female	Male
1774	14.1	5.5	6.5	8.0
1978	16.7	7.7	9.7	9.7
1982	19.6	10.5	11.0	9.2
1986	19.8	11.2	20.0	9.4
1990	13.3	6.5	13.6	9.5
1992	13.1	6.9	16.2	10.7

* Source: O'Hare and O'Connor, 1987; Health Research Board, 1997.

As Table 4 shows, overall rates are now quite similar between Dublin and Roscommon. Since 1974, rates for men in Roscommon have increased very little but rates for women have increased considerably. In Dublin, male rates appear to have increased during the early 1980s but have now reverted to 1970 levels. Female rates in Dublin are approximately twice those of male rates but there has been little change during this period. In Roscommon, male rates are still relatively high but the pattern is now in line with Dublin and elsewhere. While this could indicate underlying changes in Irish society resulting in greater similarity between rural and urban values and behaviour patterns, hospital in-patient or out-patient figures do not provide a sufficient basis for such a conclusion. The influence of such factors as developments in service provision provides an alternative and less speculative explanation for these changes. It may be concluded, however, that psychiatric morbidity, or, more particularly, utilisation of psychiatric services as a measure of expressing unhappiness, now appears to be similar in both urban and rural settings and this has probably been influenced by the increased provision of community psychiatric facilities evident from the 1980s on.

These findings are supported by a community study undertaken in the Dublin area to determine the prevalence of depression among women (Cleary, 1997). This study showed a one-year prevalence rate of 17.9% of the population at risk (women aged 18–65 years). The study was based on fairly rigid assessment procedures. Interviews, which were tape recorded, were conducted by a researcher trained in the use of the assessment instrument (the Present State Examination) (Wing *et al.*, 1974) and independently rated by a psychiatrist. This fairly high prevalence rate was accompanied by a particularly high level of service use. Over half (54%) of the women in the sample had sought treatment for psychological difficulties at some time and 28% were currently receiving treatment. All of the women categorised as 'cases' of depression had received treatment (77% were currently receiving treatment). The majority (74%) of those receiving treatment were attending general practitioner services, and this finding (i.e. that women are particularly strong users of GP services) is supported by research elsewhere (HMSO, 1995). The type of treatment received by these women was predominantly drug based. One third of the sample were taking psychotropic medication, mainly minor tranquillisers, at the time of interview. Although there appeared to be a general feeling among these women that such treatment was of doubtful efficacy, especially in the long term, very few of them questioned the prescribing of these drugs and, in general, they were unwilling to discontinue taking medication.

These findings based on community studies tend to support a gendered pattern of mental disorder in Ireland, at least in terms of service presentation. In the hospital system men predominate overall although both men and women dominate in certain diagnostic categories. These diagnostic groupings – depression and substance abuse – are generally categorised as minor psychiatric disorders and hence are more in evidence in the community services. There is a good deal of research evidence, including the available Irish research presented above, which suggests a high prevalence of depression in general practitioner services (HMSO, 1996). As women present for treatment of depression more often than men the predominance of women in this area of the health service is understandable. The pattern of treatment for substance abuse, especially alcoholism, is not so clear-cut. Since the early 1980s the public hospital system has significantly reduced the number of beds available for alcoholism treatment and this is reflected in the statistics (Keogh and Walsh, 1996). Private facilities still exist and a number of public out-patient units have been developed, but alcoholism as a category is becoming increasingly marginalised from the public psychiatric service. However, according to available statistics, men do predominate in this type of disorder. Is there a relationship between the two diagnostic categories of depression and alcoholism? There is a possibility that these diagnoses represent different culturally acceptable labels for men and women experiencing the same kinds of difficulties (Weissman and Klerman, 1977; Egeland and Hostetter, 1983). A good deal of evidence suggests that men and women manifest distress in different ways (Duncombe and Marsden, 1993). For men the expression of distress may be more outwardly-directed, and for women more inwardly-directed (Cloward and Piven, 1979). Certainly, women report more symptoms of distress than men (Newmann, 1984). There is also evidence that those who present with alcoholism often have depression or that the two conditions may correlate in families (Tyndall, 1974; Weissman and Klerman, 1977).

Data relating to suicide in Ireland provide additional information on male and female responses to distress. More men than women commit suicide in Ireland and suicide is now the second most common cause of death among men in the 15–24 year age group (Department of Health, 1996). This trend is evident throughout the western world where male suicide rates are at least twice female rates (Pritchard, 1995). Women in Ireland are less vulnerable to suicide in every age category except in the grouping 44–55 years (Department of Health, 1996). Other factors such as age and marital status are implicated in suicide rates but there is substantial evidence linking suicide and mental disorder, principally depression (Barraclough and Hughes, 1987). Why do men – particularly young men – kill themselves more frequently than women while women, in general, report more distress? One possible explanation is that men in this age group have increased access to drugs and alcohol and this, along with psychological problems, makes them more vulnerable to suicide (Hawton *et al.*,1993). The rationale here is that drugs and/or alcohol induce or compound compulsive behaviour. Gender and the method of suicide adopted are also linked in that men use more violent methods to kill themselves and are therefore more likely to succeed (McClure, 1987). Alternatively, does the fact that more men than women kill themselves at this age imply that men suffer more severe distress than women or that men are less tolerant of symptoms such as depression? Finally, more specifically social factors might be involved. Men may have less tenuous social links while women's close connection to the family network may act as a protective factor. Gender differences in help-seeking behaviour constitute another possible explanation (Foster *et al.*, 1997), although this must be considered along with other factors explaining why people in general succumb to distress.

If we consider the possible causes of depression in women and men, we encounter, as already indicated, an abundance of work on depression among women and very little in relation to men. There are a number of competing explanations from various disciplines accounting for depression in women. Traditional medical interpretations of depression in women are based on biological and/or hormonal causes but there are also various psychological and psychoanalytical definitions. Within sociology the causes of mental disorder in women are also contested. One theory links psychological disorder to the stress women encounter in their lives. This approach either concentrates on a general analysis of the female social role or examines specific stresses in the woman's life. A particular focus here is the married woman's role, since marital status is linked for women (but not for men) to psychological distress (Gove and Tudor, 1973; Radloff, 1975). Various aspects of the marital role have been examined e.g. being a full time housewife (Gove and Tudor, 1973) having young children (Brown and Harris, 1978) and working outside the home (Cochrane and Stopes-Roe, 1981). Attempts have also been made to incorporate these variables into an explanatory model of depression (Brown and Harris, 1978). Such studies have failed to isolate a general factor or set of factors and it now appears that the process is more complex than previously considered. Some studies, for example, have shown that women who work outside the home are less psychologically healthy than full-time housewives (Thoits, 1986). What appears to be central to an understanding of this process is the meaning of the role or aspect of the role to the woman (Simon, 1995). In this way, research into the factors associated with depression in Irish women reported elsewhere (Cleary, 1997) indicates that stresses or life events may be important in terms of the timing of onset of depression but do not explain adequately why a woman becomes depressed in the first place. A life span approach appears to offer more possibilities. The Dublin study (Cleary, 1997) showed that women who were depressed did have more serious difficulties both in their past and present lives. Childhood disadvantages included lack of parental care due to parental psychiatric illness, alcoholism and marital disharmony and these factors appeared to form part of a process of vulnerability. Vulnerability of itself, however, did not produce distress unless certain additional negative factors were also present, or certain positive factors, such as social support, absent. A crucial element here, as suggested, is meaning, and depression appears more likely to result if a core person or object is lost or threatened (Brown and Prudo, 1981). It may be that women are more attuned to the effects of interpersonal stress because of the way they are socialised (Rosenfield, 1980). They may also be more exposed to situations of stress because of their key position in the family network. The importance of role and meaning, however, is not confined to women. It implies that, because of the centrality of women within the home, and perhaps because of the way they have been socialised, losses in the area of interpersonal relations with resulting low self-esteem may determine women's vulnerability to depression (Cleary, 1997). An equivalent vulnerability may be seen in men where the relevant loss in a core role is often seen in relation to unemployment and loss of work (Pritchard, 1995; Nolan and Whelan, see pp. 99–111 above). A tentative explanation for depression, embracing both men and women, is that depression is a condition to which people are likely to succumb when role loss is substantial.

An important consideration in this discussion is the high prevalence of women who attend community-based, especially general practitioner, services for depression. This is firstly linked to service provision factors such as accessibility of treatment. The take-up of services increases or decreases generally according to provision of that particular type of treatment and this effect can be seen, for instance, in the statistics on alcoholism. The Irish hospital system has continued to contain a higher proportion of men from the west of Ireland because the system initially fulfilled a specific social need in rural Ireland but this containment has continued even after significant social change (O'Hare and O'Connor, 1987). Women are now using the community services because they are fulfilling a need but women are also being contained within the service. They are more frequent attendees at GP services than men because of their own and their families' requirements. They may also have more cultural flexibility in terms of expressing certain types of psychological difficulties but the expression of distress is channelled into this type of service partly because of a lack of alternatives. Finally, women are more likely to become long-term attendees because of the drug based treatment they usually receive (Cooperstock, 1976). Overall it may be said that the individualising tendencies of medical practice which focus on the presenting problem rather than the structural causes are unlikely to solve many of these women's problems.

Some sociological as well as feminist theories link mental disorder and the oppression of women in society (Showalter, 1987; Ussher, 1991). There is evidence connecting the roles and tasks of women in society to powerlessness (Radloff, 1975) and hence to depression but there is also evidence that men are affected by powerlessness in an increasingly changing economy (Nolan and Whelan, see pp. 99–111 above). Similarly feminist accounts citing the frequency of mental disorder among women as a way of regulating women are somewhat simplistic. The evidence in Ireland and elsewhere is that men and women are both regulated within the psychiatric system albeit in a different way. In fact the evidence is that men are more likely to be severely regulated (i.e. hospitalised) if their symptoms involve violence. Finally, if we examine another strand of feminist analysis i.e. that a specific sexism operates within medical discourse – there does appear to be some support for this (Broverman *et al.*,1970; Busfield 1989). Certain stereotypes of maleness and femaleness do operate within medicine and psychiatry and the prescribing of medication by GPs to women in far greater numbers than to men does appear to support this (Cooperstock, 1976).

If we draw together all of these findings we can see that a number of issues are involved. There is a gender pattern in psychiatric service usage both at hospital and community levels although the situation in Ireland is somewhat complicated by historical factors. Overall, men tend to predominate in the Irish hospital system and this has been the pattern in both the nineteenth and twentieth centuries. Women tend to predominate in the community services. This pattern is closely linked to diagnosis. In conclusion it may be said that in Ireland men and women predominate in different diagnostic categories and in different areas of the mental health landscape.

Acknowledgements

I would like to thank Dr Dermot Walsh (Health Research Board) for his permission to use unpublished data and Ms Fiona Keogh for her assistance in accessing the data.

References

Allen, H. (1987) *Justice Unbalanced: Gender, Psychiatry and Judicial Decisions*. Milton Keynes: Open University Press.

Barraclough, B.M. and J. Hughes (1987) *Suicide: Clinical and Epidemiological Studies*. London: Croom Helm.

Broverman, I.K., D.M. Broverman, F.E. Clarkson, P.S. Rosenkrantz and S.R.Vogel (1970) Sex role stereotypes and clinical judgement of mental health, *Journal of Consulting and Clinical Psychology*, 34: 1–7.

Brown, G.W. and T. Harris (1978) *The Social Origins of Depression*. London: Tavistock.

Brown, G.W. and R. Prudo (1981) Psychiatric disorder in a rural and urban population. aetiology of depression, *Psychological Medicine*, 11: 581–99.

Busfield, J. (1989) Sexism and society, *Sociology*, 23: 343–64.

Busfield, J. (1996) *Men, Women and Madness*. London: Macmillan.

Chesler, P. (1972) *Women and Madness*. New York: Doubleday.

Clark, V.A., C.S. Aneshensel, R.R. Frerichs and T.M. Morgan (1981) Analysis of effects of sex and age on response to items on the CES-D scale, *Psychiatry Research*, 5: 171–81.

Cleary, A. (1987) 'The resocialisation project: a report on the EU Rehabilitation Unit in St. Brendan's Hospital', Dublin: Eastern Health Board.

Cleary, A. (1997) Madness and mental health in Irish women, in: A.Byrne and M. Leonard (eds), *Women in Irish Society: A Sociological Reader*. Belfast: Beyond the Pale.

Cloward, R. and F.F. Piven (1979) Hidden protest: the channelling of female protest and resistance, *Signs*, 4: 651–9.

Cochrane, R. and M. Stopes-Roe (1981) Women, marriage, employment and mental health, *British Journal of Psychiatry*, 139: 373–81.

Comstock, G.W. and K.J. Helsing (1976) Symptoms of depression in two communities, *Psychological Medicine*, 6: 551–63.

Cooperstock, R. (1976) Psychotropic drug use among women, *Canadian Medical Journal Association Journal*, 115: 760–3.

Craig, T.J. and P.A. Van Natta (1979) Influence of demographic characteristics on two measures of depressive symptoms, *Archives of General Psychiatry*, 36: 149–54.

Department of Health (1996) *National Task Force on Suicide Interim Report*. Dublin: Stationery Office.

Department of Health and Social Security (1986) *Mental Health Statistics for England 1986*. London: HMSO.

Dohrenwend, B.P. and B.S. Dohrenwend (1976) Sex differences and psychiatric disorders, *American Journal of Sociology*, 81: 1447–54.

Dressler, W.W. and L.W. Badger (1985) Epidemiology of depressive symptoms in black communities: a comparative analysis, *Journal of Nervous and Mental Diseases*, 173: 212–20.

Duncombe, J. and D. Marsden (1993) Love and intimacy: the gender division of emotion work, *Sociology*, 27: 221–41.

Durkheim, E. (1951) *Suicide : A Study in Sociology*. (Translated by J.A Spaulding and G. Simpson), Glencoe, IL: Free Press.

Egeland, J.A. and A.M. Hostetter (1983) Amish Study 1: Affective disorders among the Amish, 1976–1980, *American Journal of Psychiatry*, 140: 56–61.

Ehrenreich, B. and D. English (1976) *Complaints and Disorders: The Sexual Politics of Sickness*. London: Writers and Readers Publishing Cooperative.

Faris, R. and H. Dunham (1939) *Mental Disorders in Urban Areas*. Chicago: University of Chicago Press.

Finnane, M. (1981) *Insanity and the Insane in Post-Famine Ireland*. London: Croom Helm.

Foster, T., K. Gillespie and R. McCelland, R. (1997) Mental disorders and suicide in Northern Ireland, *British Journal of Psychiatry*, 170: 447–52.

Foucault, M. (1967) *Madness and Civilisation: A History of Madness in the Age of Reason*. London: Tavistock.

Goffman, E. (1961) *Asylums*. Harmondsworth: Penguin.

Goldberg, D. and P. Huxley (1980) *Mental Illness in the Community: The Pathway to Psychiatric Care*. London: Tavistock.

Goldstein, J.M. (1992) Gender and schizophrenia: a summary of findings, *Schizophrenia Monitor*, 2: 1–4.

Gove, W.R. and J. Tudor (1973). Adult sex roles and mental illness, *American Journal of Sociology*, 77: 812–35.

Hawton, K., J. Fagg, S. Platt and M. Hawkins (1993) Factors associated with suicide after parasuicide in young people, *British Medical Journal*, 306: 1641–4.

Health Research Board (1997) Unpublished figures.

HMSO (1995) *Morbidity Statistics From General Practice: 4th National Study 1991–1992*, Series MB5 No.3, London: HMSO.

HMSO (1996) *Key Health Statistics from General Practice*. London: HMSO.

HMSO (1997) *Hospital Episode Statistics, 1994–95*, unpublished figures.

Hollingshead, A.B. and F.C. Redlich (1958) *Social Class and Mental Illness: A Community Study*. New York: Wiley.

Jenkins, R. (1985) Sex differences in minor psychiatric morbidity, *Psychological Medicine*, Monograph Supplement No 7, Cambridge: Cambridge University Press.

Keogh, F. and D. Walsh (1996) *Irish Psychiatric Hospitals and Units Activities 1995*. Dublin: Health Research Board.

Kessler, R., K. McGonagle, M. Swartz, D. Blazer and G. Nelson (1993) Sex and depression in the National Comorbidity Survey 1: lifetime prevalence, chronicity and recurrence, *Journal of Affective Disorders*, 29 (Special Issue): 85–96.

Linn, M.W., K.I. Hunter and P.R. Perry (1979). Differences by sex and ethnicity in the psychosocial adjustment of the elderly, *Journal of Health and Social Behaviour*, 20: 273–81.

McClure, G.M.S. (1987) Suicide in England and Wales 1975–84: mode of death, *British Journal of Psychiatry*, 150: 309–14.

Malcolm, E. (1989) *Swift's Hospital: A History of St. Patrick's Hospital Dublin, 1746–1989*. Dublin, Gill & Macmillan.

Moran, R. and D. Walsh (1992) *The Irish Psychiatric Hospitals and Units Census 1992*. Dublin: Health Research Board.

Myers, S.K., M.M. Wiseman, G.L. Tichsler, C.E.Holzer, P.J. Leaf, H. Orvasihel, J.C. Anthony, J.H. Boyd, J.D. Burke, M. Kramer and R. Stoltzman (1984) Six-month prevalence of psychiatric disorders in three communities, 1980 to 1982, *Archives of General Psychiatry*, 41: 959–67.

Newmann, J.P. (1984) Sex differences in symptoms of depression: clinical disorder or normal distress? *Journal of Health and Social Behaviour*, 25: 136–59.

Ní Nualláin, M., A.O'Hare, D.Walsh, B. Blake, J.V. Halpenny and P.F. O'Brien, (1984) The incidence of mental illness in Ireland – patients contacting psychiatric services in three Irish counties, *Irish Journal of Psychiatry*, 5: 23–9.

O'Hare, A. and A. O'Connor (1987) Gender differences in treated mental illness in the Republic of Ireland, in: C. Curtin, P. Jackson and B. O'Connor (eds) *Gender in Irish Society*. Galway: Galway University Press.

Orley, J.H. and J.K.Wing (1979) Psychiatric disorders in two African villages, *Archives of General Psychiatry*, 36: 513–20.

Parker, G. (1979) Sex differences in non-clinical depression: review and assessment of previous studies, *Australian and New Zealand Journal of Psychiatry*, 13: 127–32.

Penfold, P.S. and G.A.Walker (1984) *Women and the Psychiatric Paradox*. Milton Keynes: Open University Press.

Pritchard, C. (1995) *Suicide – The Ultimate Rejection? A Psychosocial Study*. Buckingham: Open University Press.

Radloff, L. (1975) Sex differences in depression: the effects of occupation and marital status, *Sex Roles*, 1: 249–65.

Robins, J. (1986) *Fools and Mad: A History of the Insane in Ireland*. Dublin: Institute of Public Administration.

Rosenfield, S. (1980) Sex differences in depression: Do women always have higher rates? *Journal of Health and Social Behaviour*, 21: 33–42.

Showalter, E. (1987) *The Female Malady*. London: Virago.

Simon, R.W. (1995) Gender, multiple roles, role meaning and depression, *Journal of Health and Social Behaviour*, 36: 182–94.

Smith, D. (1975) The statistics on mental illness: what they will not tell us about women and why, in: D. Smith and S. David (eds) *Women Look at Psychiatry*. Vancouver: Press Gang.

Szasz, T. (1961) *The Myth of Mental Illness*. New York: Hoeber-Harper.

Thoits, P. (1986) Multiple identities: examining gender and marital status differences in distress, *American Sociological Review*, 51: 259–72.

Tyndall, M. (1974) Psychiatric study of 1000 alcoholic patients, *Canadian Psychiatric Association Journal*, 19: 21–4.

Ussher, J. (1991) *Women's Madness: Misogyny or Mental Illness?* London: Harvester Wheatsheaf.

Wing, J.K., J.E. Cooper and N. Sartorius (1974) *Measurement and Classification of Psychiatric Symptoms: An Instruction Manual for the PSE and Catego Program*. Cambridge: Cambridge University Press.

Weissman, M.M., R. Bland, P. Joyce, S. Newman, E.Wells and H-U. Wittchen (1993) Sex differences in rates of depression: cross-national perspectives, *Journal of Affective Disorders*, 29 (Special Issue): 77–84.

Weissman, M.M. and Klerman, G.L. (1977) Sex differences in the epidemiology of depression, *Archives of General Psychiatry*, 34: 98–111.

13

The Asylum In Ireland:
A Brief Institutional History and Some
Local Effects

A. Jamie Saris

> Alas! The only truly impressive thing in Cork I remembered, as the train rolled in, is its lunatic asylum. It is remarkable even for Ireland, a sparsely populated land where only the pious and unhinged assemble in any number – Honor Tracy, *Mind You I've Said Nothing* (1953: 115).

Introduction

In the last thirty years, the anthropological and sociological literature on the Asylum (and the sciences that developed within it) has grown enormously. These works cover several theoretical approaches and national traditions. Amongst the best-known authors who have studied this topic are Foucault (1973), Castel (1976), Charuty (1985), and Jodelet (1989) for France; Drwyer (1987), Grob (1992, 1994), Rothman (1985), Tomes (1984) and Goffman (1961) for America; Porter (1987a, 1987b), Skultans (1975, 1979), Scull (1979, 1981, 1984), Ramon (1990), and the contributors to Berrios and Freeman (1991) in England; and Fisher (1985) for the Caribbean. The two main books on the history of the mental hospital system in Ireland are Finnane (1981) and Robins (1986).[1]

The asylum in Ireland is interesting for a number of reasons. Irish asylum population figures, for example, rose very rapidly in the nineteenth century, particularly when measured against declining population figures for the island in the post-Famine period.

Well into the twentieth century, the relatively high numbers of inpatients in Irish mental hospitals led to several theories about the susceptibility of 'the Irish' to various forms of pathological irrationality (e.g., World Health Organisation, 1973). The peculiarities of Irish culture (Scheper-Hughes, 1982) to viruses in sheep's brains (Torrey *et al.*, 1984) have been mentioned as

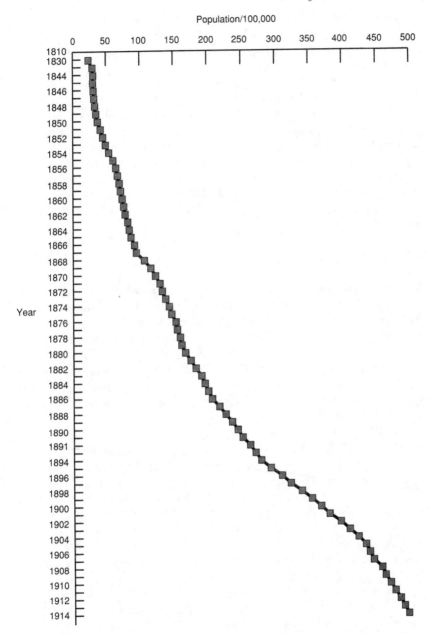

POPULATION/100,000 IN RESIDENCE IN IRISH DISTRICT LUNATIC
ASYLUMS, 1830–1915 (Adapted from Finnane, 1981: Appendix F,
with Returns from Lunatic Asylums (Ireland) 1830, 1840)

possible bad influences, though in recent years, this association has been fiercely attacked (Clare, 1991, also the other contributors to Keane, 1991).

Before these theories, the imputed association between Ireland and 'lunacy' had also served the bombast of the apologist for the British colonial subjugation of Ireland, the vision of the comic writer interested in demonstrating the quaintness of the Irish, and the rhetoric of the nationalist committed to showing the damages inflicted by British rule. Such diverse figures as Prime Minister Gladstone, who saw the relief of lunatics as one of the main benefits accruing from the disestablishment of the Church of Ireland (cited in Finnane, 1981: 55–7), and the Nationalist parliamentarian John Redmond, who pointed to the large number of Irish interned in lunatic asylums as evidence that 'Under your [English] rule it has been the survival of the unfittest in Ireland' (Redmond, 1906: 183), could accept that medical irrationality possessed the status of an Irish problem.

Studying the Asylum

Crudely, literature on the Asylum can be divided into two main approaches. Some authors argue that serious mental illnesses have afflicted humanity (perhaps in a greater or lesser degree) in all places and in all times, and that the asylum, whatever its imperfections, was a progressive response to a self-evident problem (see among others Roth and Kroll, 1986; Grob, 1994; and Rothman, 1990; for critique see Warner, 1985). Other authors are less interested in mental illness as such and much more concerned with the historical and social novelty of these (very often extraordinary) structures purpose-built to confine and rehabilitate the mad.

The development of the asylum in Ireland cannot be understood unless one appreciates both these arguments, that is to say, the growth of the Irish asylum system is inseparable from the particular social dynamics of the early nineteenth-century colonial state *and* the emergence of specialised modes of treating the insane throughout the world. Similarly, their current decay is incomprehensible without understanding how the social and medical ways of dealing with the insane have transformed internationally and the nature of Ireland's relationship to such trends.

To approach such issues, my own research centres on the cultural and historical relationships between a (recently) large mental hospital in the west of Ireland, St Columba's Hospital in Sligo town, and a market town and its environs (about 1,600 people) within the two counties (Sligo and Leitrim) served by this institution. For the purposes of this study, I call this market town *Kilronan*.

Kilronan possesses a long-standing association with the mental hospital in Sligo town that dates back to the institution's construction during the Great Hunger at the end of 1840s. Currently, the town and its environs have a quickly developing community psychiatric infrastructure that is absorbing individuals once housed in the asylum back into 'the community'. These attributes of Kilronan give us the opportunity to understand how local knowledge of disordered persons is situated within complex institutional and historical relationships (Saris, 1994, 1996).

A Short History of the Asylum

Traditional accounts of the development of the Asylum stress the cruel nature of the haphazard services for the insane before their treatment was put on a scientific basis (e.g., Robins, 1986: 23–41; Roth and Kroll, 1986, among many others). In this vision, the conquest of the asylum by medicine was an important step forward for the humane treatment of vulnerable individuals. The archetypal image that comes to us from such work is that of Philippe Pinel striking the chains off the lunatics at Bicêtre at the time of the French Revolution.

According to Pinel's own account, before he arrived on the scene all was dark and disordered in the treatment of the insane. Discarding his prejudices about such individuals, Pinel embarked on a project of cataloguing the phenomenon without biases. The data gathered formed the basis for new hypotheses, better (and more humane) treatment, and, last but not least, a scholarly tract in which the new knowledge was to be disseminated (Pinel, 1809). The narrative is a worn one, but none the worse in Pinel's hands, charting the heroic, but modestly presented, struggle of one man against a sea of ignorance and superstition.

The main tools in this struggle, according to Pinel, is the building itself, the skills and knowledge of the moral manager of the institution (in this case Pinel), and the abilities of its staff, all of which affect the moral and physical well-being of a patient. The moral manager, then, is a powerful but humane figure. He is in absolute control of his institution, but he also should know all those under him by name. He is stern enough to keep his staff in line and dominate the wills of his more intractable charges, but he is also approachable enough to maintain an agreeable atmosphere in the hospital, one that could cheer up even the most melancholic individual.

The idea of looking after what we would now call the mental health needs of a national population also grew out of systems of *public* hospitals that developed over Europe and North America (and to a lesser extent in other places) at about the same time that Pinel's ideas were being diffused. Following Pinel, these new asylum managers argued that categories like 'lunatic' needed to be organised according to scientific nosologies and treated accordingly (Donnelly, 1983). This led to yet another consequence – that the Asylum became increasingly professionalised. As the nineteenth century progressed lay managers gave way to physicians, and variations of the post, 'Asylum

Superintendent', became a recognised medical specialty in Europe and the United States. Fundamentally, those who financed and ran these new hospitals understood these institutions as technologies, tools able to ameliorate an important category of human affliction.

The Birth of the Asylum in Ireland

Much of this general history is relevant for Ireland's experience of the asylum. The oldest asylum for the insane on the island is St Patrick's Hospital, which was founded at the bequest of Dean Swift in 1729, and which opened its doors in 1745.[2] Swift was touched by the plight of indigents whom he considered insane, and he believed that a serious but limited problem of lunacy existed in Ireland. Thus, his will states that, if the 140-odd places provided by the bequest were not needed by 'lunatics and idiots', then vacant beds could be filled by persons with other infirmaries. Several charitable and privately-run hospitals, wards in locally-run Houses of Industry, even portions of bridewells and gaols, catering for 'lunatics and idiots', also developed in the eighteenth century, culminating in the first public hospital in Ireland for the care of the insane, the Richmond Asylum (now St Brendan's), which opened in 1817.

Tellingly, before the waves of institution-building that marked Ireland between the 1820s and 1870s, the connection between 'the Irish' (particularly those in remote parts of the island) and 'insanity' is only weakly developed. The then-popular understanding of madness (at least in Britain) saw it as a prototypical disease of *civilisation*, the result of mental strain associated with the complexity of modern living. In such a model, we would expect to find less 'insanity' in largely rural Ireland than in increasingly urban England. As *late* as 1828, for example, Andrew Halliday, the famed English asylum reformer, argued

> [T]he finer the organs of the mind have become by their greater development or their better cultivation . . . the more easily they are disordered. [Thus,] the contented peasantry of the Welsh mountains, the Western Hebrides, and the wilds of Ireland are almost free of this complaint. [Halliday, 1828: 80]

The growth of a true, centrally coordinated and inspected *system* of asylums in Ireland seemed to change these impressions. This system grew out of a Parliamentary Select Committee meeting in 1815–1816. Despite real political differences between some of the members, almost all of them warned that lunacy was on the march amongst the poorer classes on the island, particularly in the remote, ill-administered parts of the country. Furthermore, they insisted that lunacy was connected to a collection of other disorders – of space, of work, of society, of people, and relationships between persons – that also required attention.

To this end, Thomas Rice (later Baron Monteagle) gave the following testimony to the committee, refracting a set of 'well-known' attributes of the Irish peasant through an emerging medical understanding of lunacy.

[Lunacy] is an hereditary malady and therefore likely to be extended. It is connected with scrofulous habits, also hereditary and therefore advances on a double principle. It is connected with the habits of the lower classes of people in Ireland who addict themselves to the use of ardent spirits; and it is connected also with the use of Mercury. These four causes are, *a priori*, sufficient to show that it is on the increase. [*Report of the Select Committee to Consider the State of the Lunatic Poor in Ireland*, 1817: 21]

With the exception of the reference to mercury, these are durable colonial images about 'the Irish' (bad habits, genetic dysfunction, and a fatal attraction to whiskey) that have survived in one form or another even into the late twentieth century (e.g., Murphy 1975). This list of 'handicaps' also resonates with descriptions of other populations who, for one reason or another, have been marginalised in different parts of the world.

The committee then went on to trace some of the implications of this disorder for understanding life and suffering in rural Ireland. Thus, Denis Browne, a magistrate from County Mayo, could paint the following poignant, almost lyrical, picture of lunacy among the rural poor.[3]

There is nothing so shocking as madness in the cabin of a peasant, where the man is out laboring in the fields for his bread, and the care of the woman of the house is scarcely sufficient for the attendance of the children. When a strong man or woman gets the complaint, the only way they have to manage is by making a hole in the floor of the cabin for the person with a crib over it to prevent his getting up, the hole is generally five feet deep, and they give the wretched being his food there, and there he generally dies. Of all human calamity, I know of none equal to this in the country parts of Ireland which I am acquainted with. [*Report of the Select Committee to Consider the State of the Lunatic Poor in Ireland* 1817: 23]

Here, madness is situated both in the retarded productive capacity of the peasant household (the people pictured here are barely keeping up) and the confused space that they inhabit (all the action in the vignette takes place in a one room cabin). In this fashion, Browne sketches a portrait of a population that is at once helpless and dangerous, and he implies that the amelioration of lunacy in Ireland will require a multi-level reorganisation of space, time, and person.

The Asylum System in Nineteenth-Century Ireland

Legislation following the publication of the report of the 1817 Committee resulted in the construction of seven new hospitals (and the conversion of three others) into the Irish District Lunatic Asylum System in the 1820s. London and Dublin Castle hit upon a novel way of funding such institutions that exempted these reformers, many of whom sat on their local Grand Juries, from fiscal accountability. It also fitted in nicely with the endemic centralisation that marked the governance of Ireland in the nineteenth century. Briefly, Dublin Castle would force the respective counties in a particular district to take a loan from the Consolidated Fund, which would then be paid back out of the rates over the course of twenty years. This funding mechanism was different from that found in the sister kingdom, which made such a loan only on the voluntary petition of the county concerned, a situation that was not to change until the 1840s when something very like the Irish model was developed for England and Wales (see MacDonagh, 1977 and Porter, 1987a).

The asylum system was also the first moment of a profound bureaucratic movement in Ireland. The Royal Irish Constabulary, for example, is only constituted as a island-wide paramilitary body in 1833 (Broeker, 1970). A National School system is begun in 1834 to educate the young *in English* throughout the island. The Ordnance Survey attempts to completely map and name in English every point in Ireland, an exercise in domination that is brilliantly explored in Brian Friel's play *Translations* (for a strong critique of Friel, see Anderson, 1975). Finally a full, nationally administered Workhouse system is begun in 1838 replacing the old Houses of Industries administered by local corporations (Feingold, 1984). By the middle part of the century a devotional revolution in the Catholic Church (Larkin, 1972) was also under way, moving daily Irish practices towards more recognisably 'civil' (read British) lines (see Inglis, 1987). All these changes involved a profound transformation of person, place, and rationality in Ireland.

The Famine and the District Lunatic Asylum System

The seeming necessity for these asylums also quickly dovetailed into a set of images that went well beyond the confinement and transformation of a limited number of deviants. As they began to fill and overflow, for example, more committees were called in to investigate the issue. The Select Committee of 1843 admitted from the outset that,

> Although the accommodation provided in the ten district Asylums very considerably exceeds that which was contemplated by the Committee of 1817, it is very far from meeting the necessities of the case. [*Report of the Select Committee to Consider the State of the Lunatic Poor in Ireland*, 1843: iii]

After taking more evidence, the committee suggested that seven more hospitals be built. By the time the tenders for these buildings were awarded, the Famine was raging in much of the island.

The local situation in the counties of Sligo and Leitrim give some sense for the various levels of meaning that the Asylum condensed for Ireland. The Liberal, later to be Nationalist, *Sligo Champion*, for example, was delighted with the new asylum project in Sligo town on strictly fiscal grounds. In two short paragraphs, they congratulated the local architect whose tender had been accepted and they briefly noted the anticipated cost of the place – £33,000, an impressive figure for the time. The Conservative, Orange *Sligo Journal* made essentially identical points concerning the relief that such a public building would afford the hard-pressed region, but saw broader issues that the building of an institution of this nature raised.

> A dearth of work now generally prevails and this extensive building will most timely occupy many deserving tradesmen and labourers, who have long suffered from the pinching gripe of idleness; their peaceful demeanour when pining under the scourge of famine has rebounded to their credit. The visitations of an All-Wise Providence have been born by Connaughtmen with a fortitude fully becoming and heroic: their endurance of accumulated misery has been lauded from the judicial bench and elsewhere, but the precious reward of well-doing can alone be dispensed by the Kings of Kings, who is now and at all times allotting to his creatures whatever is just and right. Chastisement rather than indulgence, in our sphere of wickedness is conducive to the spread of penitence and Christianity. The Earth is at this present instant groaning with good gifts from on High, the fruit of which, it is ardently hoped, the labourious classes will tranquilly enjoy in due season. Meantime they must be watchful, sober and thrifty – in a word our peasantry ought to guard against evil-doers; the clamorous and turbulent must be kept within the bounds of propriety, in regard to this much abused country, whose prosperity has been so cruelly retarded by idle factions. The rich treasures of Ireland can best be secured by casting aside discord and pulling together in amity (*Sligo Journal*, 25 August 1848).

The author of the *Sligo Journal* article uses the institution-to-be to invoke a variety of images of restraint ('peaceful demeanour', 'penitence and Christianity', and 'bounds of propriety') and pleads for tranquillity from its local 'laborious classes' while nervously acknowledging their potential for disorder at this time of 'accumulated misery'. He looks upon the building as part providential salvation and part index of dangerous times. While he is clearly relieved by the economic support that the construction of such an institution will undoubtedly provide, in his tone, he seems far from certain that even after the asylum is built all 'the clamorous and turbulent' will be found on the inside of its walls.

Official Despair

This second wave of asylums filled up even faster than the first one. In only fourteen years, the Sligo-Leitrim institution quietly surpassed its official capacity. This cycle of overflow and expansion was repeated throughout the island. In this fashion, the limited problem confronted and (presumably solved) by the Committee of 1817 became increasingly complex and convoluted, and, slowly, an initial discourse of 'reform' shaded into a much less ambitious rhetoric of merely keeping up with the problem. Thus, another wave of asylums were duly commissioned in the late 1860s with much the same results. If, by the middle of the nineteenth century, the original assessments for the control of the problem of lunacy in Ireland began to seem optimistic, then, by the late 1800s the continued growth of these institutions became an issue of great official and medical concern (e.g., Corbett, 1874). Indeed, from 1880 to 1893 alone, the number of lunatics in Irish asylums increased by 33% in absolute terms. Because of immigration, however, the ratio per 100,000 of lunatics in asylums to the general population increased by almost 50% (*Special Report From the Inspectors of the Lunatics to the Chief Secretary on the Alleged Increasing Prevalence of Insanity in Ireland*, 1894: 6).

This rhetoric of hope for the Asylum beginning in the initial decades of the century and its subsequent disillusionment after the Famine bears some striking parallels with other discourses. The century begins, for example, with many elements of the Penal Laws still on the books and closes with a concerted attempt to 'kill Home Rule with kindness'. Ultimately, these initiatives failed according to the standards under which they were brought into being, that is, to coerce Ireland into submitting to, or conciliate her into accepting, her status in the empire. This failure tended to imbue the problems of Ireland with an aura of intractability. The asylum's struggle with a never-ending burden of 'incurables', therefore, fit into a much broader picture of obstinate 'Irish problems' and increasingly impotent British government responses that were locked together in mutually developing embrace.

Perhaps there is no better measure of the increasing bureaucratic momentum of the asylum system, than the difference between the sizes of the first and last official British Parliamentary reports on lunacy in the nineteenth century. The document produced by the Committee of 1817, for example, measured a slim 54 pages. In it, the Committee reviewed *all* the evidence brought before it and outlined several recommendations they deemed necessary to rationally address, and ultimately to *solve*, the problem. The Committee of 1890–91 required over 100 pages merely to *introduce* the issues surrounding the District Lunatic Asylum system in Ireland. It filled two heavy volumes with the copious amount of evidence brought before the commissioners. Far from talking in terms of solving the problem once and for all, this committee sought merely to render it more manageable.

The Irish Asylum in the Twentieth Century

It is important to note here that within the broader context of Europe and America, many of the dynamics of the filling up of Irish asylums are recognisable. Most Western countries have experimented with the specific confinement of 'lunacy', and they have seen their initially circumscribed problem and institutional response grow and expand. Ultimately, they have all experienced something that can justifiably be labelled the 'Great Disillusionment', a moving away from the idea that mass confinement as such can be rendered cost-effective, morally palatable, *and* therapeutic or rehabilitative. Scull's observations (1979, 1981) about the forces of 'reform' in the English experience – that they marshalled in the camp of the asylum in the nineteenth century, while they expressed profound reservations about it in the twentieth – is broadly applicable across America and Europe, including Ireland.

Ireland is interesting, though, because of both the relative size that such institutions attained and the resonances that they held for external perceptions of the island. By the early twentieth century, Limerick, for example, interned nearly one per cent of the county on the grounds of the mental hospital (Dawson, 1911). It is scarcely surprising, therefore, that Honor Tracy, cited in the opening quote, could casually point to the importance of the mental hospital for 'the Irish'. She is but one example (and more palatable than many) of a venerable tradition of popular writers who have made this connection between 'irrationality' and 'Ireland' for the English-speaking world (e.g., Hammerton, 1900; for overview, see Lebow, 1976: ch.1–3 and Curtis, 1984; among many others).

The issue of whether or not there was substantially more *insanity* in Ireland than in other countries during this or any other time is, on the other hand, quite difficult. Any answer is fraught with assumptions that are untestable. Some researchers, for example, have tried to show that certain diagnostic categories which tend to require long-term hospitalisation, such as schizophrenia, were at one time over-used in Ireland (Dean *et al.*, 1972). Such work neglects the history of the term 'schizophrenia' (it was only coined by Breuler at the end of the nineteenth century), and it ignores the profound changes that have occurred in psychiatric diagnostic categories in recent years (compare 'schizophrenia' in *Diagnostic and Statistical Manual of Mental Disorders*-II to *Diagnostic and Statistical Manual of Mental Disorders*-IV).

What we can say with some degree of certainty is that by the 1960s Irish psychiatry began to express profound discomfort with how asylum-based was the profession. By this time, the Republic of Ireland had 6.6 asylum in-patients/1,000 of the population, more than twice the figure for the United States (Department of Health, 1966: 17–23; also Walsh, 1968). Since the 1950s, however, particularly in the United States, asylum populations had started to dwindle. A variety of reasons are mentioned as a cause of this slow decline. First, serious mental illnesses, such as the family of schizophrenias, had by then became the target of drug therapy. Largactil (or Thorazine as it was called in the US) had dramatic effects on *some* psychotic patients, allowing them to lead lives outside of the mental hospital. Such drug therapy has enjoyed gradual improvement since that time. Second, as the 1960s progressed and the in-patient population decline continued apace, more and more Western countries began to worry about the deteriorating conditions of these predominantly nineteenth-century buildings. In particular, policy-makers expressed concern about the cost of bringing these structures up to modern building standards. Finally, a general social movement, encompassing some psychiatrists and academics, but, more importantly, individuals who had hitherto been constituted as psychiatric subjects (such as homosexuals to people who had spent much of their lives in asylums) both challenged the legitimacy of some psychiatric knowledge and focused public attention on the enormously stigmatising quality of committal to a mental hospital (Tantam, 1991). Far from thinking of the asylum as a sort of factory manufacturing productive citizens, this grimmer version of the institution saw it as a kind of warehouse, inferior accommodation for damaged persons whom society did not want (e.g., Goffman, 1961). A broad political consensus, encompassing such diverse elements as policy-makers interested in reducing the profile of 'big government' and utopian visionaries valorising the 'community' as a place of refuge from a heartless 'society', formed around the proposition that the time had come to close down these big institutions (Bassuk and Gerson, 1978; Scull 1984; Bennett, 1991; among many others).

This process, widely known as *deinstitutionalisation*, quickened dramatically in Britain and the United States during the 1970s, followed in short order by Italy, then France, and, eventually, Ireland. All these countries had been experiencing gradually declining in-patient populations, but now the emptying began in earnest, very often with little sense for what was to come after the extinction of the large hospitals (for critiques of this process, see Isaac and Armat, 1990; Scull, 1984; Fadden *et al.*, 1987 among many others). The result of these changes in Ireland is that the large buildings scattered across the countryside that filled up at such a furious pace in the 1800s, now stand empty or all but empty at the end of the twentieth century. Only 25 years ago, for example, St Columba's Mental Hospital was the third largest population centre in the two counties it served. Now, the Old Building is locked tight, awaiting either some other use or condemned to fall slowly into ruins. The last working unit of the hospital grounds is currently slated for transfer to the recently enlarged General Hospital.

Kilronan and the Decline of the Irish Asylum

Nonetheless, just as the construction of such institutions had local effects, so too do their current dispersal and transformation. Consider the seemingly straightforward decision of the Health Service to make Kilronan the centre for a new regime of 'community' psychiatry. When the Irish mental hospital service deinstitutionalised in earnest according to an imported French model of 'sectors' (*Planning For the Future*, 1984), they cast about for obvious 'centres' wherein to coordinate these area activities. As often as not, they settled on older command-control points from a colonial past. Kilronan was just such a spot.

Kilronan was established as a strong point by Anglo-Normans worried about the hostile countryside that was the north of Connacht in the early fourteenth century. In the middle of the confiscated lands of one of the more important clans in this region, an earl built a castle, not far from an abbey patronised by the old owners of the district. The developing village that survived the castle's demise in the 1600s seemed like a logical place for an 'improving' landlord to situate one of the most modern flax mills in Ireland in the middle of the eighteenth century. And, about eighty years after that, Dublin felt that it would make a good site for a railway station because, by that time, Kilronan was an economic centre in its own right. Ironically, the town's history of social, political and economic importance eventually contributed to its developing reputation as a 'mental illness blackspot' in the twentieth century, as record-keeping became more routinised and new aetiological theories diffused into the area through the professional class that ran the institution. Inmates, then patients, and then clients (as psychiatric terminology changed), from well outside the town, had long listed Kilronan as their address, an administrative epitaph to fading local importance, but now a marker of a serious problem. During this process, however, the site for the production of all this knowledge was itself transforming, from the Sligo-Leitrim District Lunatic Asylum to St Columba's Mental Hospital to a decaying core of a new regime of community psychiatry, culminating in the official closure of the Old Building in the early 1990s. Still, well after almost all of Kilronan's pretensions to being a centre had largely vanished, it was chosen as a 'logical' place to house a day hospital and three group hostels because the older generation of locals, who were now senior nurses and administrators in charge of running down and replacing the asylum, remembered the earlier importance of the town.

This decision has already had real (if no doubt unintended) effects. There is certainly some connection, for example, between town's recent 'revival' and the situating of the new 'community' psychiatric institutions in and near it. To be sure, the economic situation in the Republic of Ireland has much improved in recent years, but the infusion of cash and custom that the day hospital and hostels represents at the very least cannot have harmed this local recovery. On average thirty people a day use this service from Monday through Friday. According to my calculations, based on tallying individual expenditures for items like sweets and alcohol and estimating Health Board expenditures for providing dinner and tea for the clients, this population is directly responsible for upwards of £400/week of direct trade in the town. This figure *does not* include the more than £300,000 that has been spent in and around the town over the course of the last several years in fixed capital costs, nor does it take into account the occasional sizable purchase that one of the 'deinstitutionalised' clients makes after careful husbanding of his or her Disabled Persons Maintenance Allowance (DPMA). Far from ending, then, the association between a mental hospital and a community seems to have entered another historical moment.

Conclusion

From the relatively easy access that the recently 'deinstitutionalised' enjoy to the town and its amenities to the largely untroubled tone of the relationship between the townspeople, the clients, and the formal health services, the programme in and around Kilronan is quite faithful to the vision of the winding down of the large district mental hospitals and the 'community treatment' of the mentally ill offered in Irish government policy documents (e.g., The Psychiatric Services, 1984). At this level, the process of deinstitutionalisation in the Sligo–Leitrim area at least must be counted a success. This success will remain dependent on the continuing state financial support for the new regime of community psychiatry. It will also be dependent on how a long-standing institutional relationship between a mental hospital and a community survives the transformation of both its constituent elements.

Notes

I am indebted to Siobhán Kerr and David Slattery for assistance in preparing Graph I.

[1] See also, Harris (1930) and Kirkpatrick (1934) for useful data on the history and function of the Irish District Lunatic Asylum System.

[2] Satirising this bequest, Jonathan Swift wrote in the amusing poem, 'Verses on the Death of Dr Swift',

> He gave the little wealth he had
> To build a house for fools and mad
> To show by one satiric touch
> No nation needed it so much.

[3] If the importance of a quote can be judged from the frequency of its citation, then Browne's testimony is very important indeed. It is cited approvingly in the Introductions of the Reports of the commissions of 1843, 1879, and 1890–91. It becomes a critical image of the suffering of the 'insane' in nineteenth-century Ireland, a place that, if 'suffering' could somehow be quantified and scaled, had any number of images that might have attracted as much official sympathy.

References

Anderson, John Harwood (1975) *A Paper Landscape: The Ordinance Survey in Nineteenth-Century Ireland*. Oxford: Claredon Press.

Bassuk, Ellen L. and Samuel Gerson (1978) Deinstitutionalization and mental health services, *Scientific American*, 238(2): 46–53.

Bennett, D. (1991) The drive towards community, in: Berrios, G. and Freeman, H. (eds) *150 Years of British Psychiatry*. London: Gaskell.

Berrios, G. and H. Freeman (eds) (1991) *150 Years of British Psychiatry*. London: Gaskell.

Broeker, Galen (1970) *Rural Disorder and Police Reform in Ireland, 1812–1836*. London: Routledge.

Castel, Robert (1976) *L'Ordre Psychiatrique*. Paris: Les Editions de Minuit.

Charuty, G. (1985) *Le Couvent Des Fous: L'interment et ses Usages en Languedoc aux XIXe et XXe siècles*. Paris: Flammarion.

Clare, Anthony (1991) The mad Irish? in: Keane, C. (ed.) *Mental Health in Ireland*. Dublin: Gill & Macmillan and Radio Telefis Éireann.

Corbett, W. (1874) On the statistics of insanity, past and present, *Journal of the Statistical and Social Inquiry Society of Ireland*, 6: 382–94.

Curtis, L. Perry, Jr (1971) *Apes and Angels: The Image of the Irishman in Victorian Caricature*. Washington, D.C.: Smithsonian Institute Press.

Dawson, W. R. (1911) The presidential address on the relation between the geographical distribution of insanity and that of certain social and other conditions in Ireland, *Journal of Mental Science*, 57: 538–97.

Department of Health (1966) *Commission of Inquiry on Mental Illness*. Dublin: Stationery Office.

Dean, G., J. Shea, L. Hannissy, B. Blake, and J. Halpenny (1972) A retrospective study of first admissions of young people to psychiatric hospitals in Galway, Roscommon, and Carlow, *Journal of the Irish Medical Association*, 65(22):555–60.

Diagnostic and Statistical Manual of Mental Disorders – II Edition. New York: American Psychiatric Association.

Diagnostic and Statistical Manual of Mental Disorders – IV Edition. New York: American Psychiatric Association.

Donnelly, Michael (1983) *Managing the Mind: A Study of Medical Psychology in Early Nineteenth-Century Britain.* London: Tavistock.

Drwyer, E. (1987) *Homes For the Mad.* New Brunswick, NJ: Rutgers University Press

Fadden, G., P. Bebbington, and L. Kupiers (1987) The burden of care: the impact of functional psychiatric illness on the patient's family, *British Journal of Psychiatry*, 150: 285–92.

Feingold, William L. (1984) *The Revolt of the Tenantry: the Transformation of Local Government in Ireland, 1872–1886.* Boston: Northeastern University Press.

Finnane, Mark (1981) *Insanity and the Insane in Post-Famine Ireland.* London: Croom Helm.

Fisher, Lawernce (1985) *Colonial Madness: Mental Health in the Barbadian Social Order.* New Brunswick, NJ: Rutgers University Press,

Foucault, Michel (1967) *Madness and Civilization: A History of Madness in the Age of Reason.* London: Tavistock.

Friel, Brian (1981) *Translations.* London: Faber & Faber.

Goffman, Erving (1961) *Asylums.* New York: Harmondsworth.

Grob, Gerald (1992) Mental health policy in america: myths and realities.*Health Affairs*, Fall 1992: 7–22.

Grob, Gerald (1994) *The Mad Among Us.* Boston: The Free Press.

Halliday, Andrew (1828) *A General View of the Present State of Lunatics and Lunatic Asylums.* London.

Hammerton, J.A. (ed.) (1900) *Mr Punch's Irish Humour in Picture and Story.* London: Carmelite House.

Harris, L. (1930) *A Treatise of the Law and Practice in Lunacy in Ireland.* Dublin: Corrigan and Wilson.

Inglis, T. (1991) The struggle for control of the Irish body: state, church, and society in nineteenth-century Ireland, in: Wolf, E. (ed.) *Religious Regimes and State Formation.* Albany: State University of New York Press.

Isaac, R and V. Armat (1990) *Madness in the Streets: How Psychiatry and the Law Abandoned the Mentally Ill.* New York: Free Press.

Jodelet, Denise (1989) *Folies et Représentations Sociales.* Presses Universitaires de France.

Keane, C. (ed.) (1991) *Mental Health in Ireland.* Dublin: Gill and Macmillan and Radio Telefis Éireann.

Kirkpatrick, T. (1934) *A Note on the Care of the Insane in Ireland.* Dublin: University Press.

Larkin, Emmet (1972) The devotional revolution in Ireland. *American Historical Review*, 77: 625–52.

Lebow, R.N. (1976) *White Britain and Black Ireland: The Influence of Stereotypes on Colonial Policy.* Philadelphia: Institute For the Study of Human Issues.

MacDonagh, Oliver (1977) *Ireland: The Union and its Aftermath.* London: George Allen & Unwin.

Murphy, H.B.M. (1975) Alcoholism and schizophrenia in the Irish: a review, *Transcultural Psychiatric Research Review*, 9: 116–39.

Pinel, Philippe (1809) *Traite Medico-Philosophique sur l'alienation Mentale, 2. ed., entièrement refondue et très-augmentée.* Paris: J.A. Brosson.

Poor Law Union and Lunacy Inquiry Commission (Ireland), Reports and Evidence, with Minutes and Appendices. (1879) Dublin: Alexander Thom.

Porter, Roy (1987a) *A Social History of Madness: The World Through The Eyes of the Insane.* New York: Weidenfeld & Nicolson.

Porter, Roy (1987b) *Mind-Forg'd Manacles: A History of Madness in England from the Restoration to the Regency.* Cambridge: Harvard University Press.

The Psychiatric Services (1984) *Planning For the Future.* Dublin: The Stationery Office.

Ramon, Shulamit (1985) *Psychiatry in Britain: Meaning and Policy.* London: Croom Helm.

Redmond, John (1906) *Hansard, 4th Series.* 19 February, 152: 179–94.

Report of the Select Committee to Consider the State of the Lunatic Poor in Ireland, with Minutes and Appendices. (1817) Dublin: Alexander Thom.

Report of the Select Committee to Consider the State of the Lunatic Poor in Ireland, with Minutes of Evidence, Appendices, and Index. (1843) Dublin: Alexander Thom.

Report of the Commissioners of Inquiry into the State of the Lunatic Asylums and other Institutions for the Custody and treatment of the Insane in Ireland, with Minutes and Appendices, Command 2436 XXVII 2 Vols. (1857–58). Dublin: Alexander Thom.

Robins, Joseph (1986) *Fools and Mad: A History of the Insane in Ireland.* Dublin: Institute for Public Administration.

Roth, M. and J. Kroll (1986) *The Reality of Mental Illness.* Cambridge: Cambridge University Press.

Rothman, David (1990) *The Discovery of the Asylum: Social Order and Disorder in the New Republic, Revised Edition.* Boston: Little Brown.

Saris, A. Jamie (1996) Mad kings, proper houses and an asylum in rural Ireland, *American Anthropologist,* 98(3): 539–54.

Saris, A. Jamie (1994) 'The Proper Place For Lunatics: Asylum, Person, and History in a Rural Irish Community', Unpublished doctoral dissertation, University of Chicago.

Scheper-Hughes, Nancy (1982) *Saints, Scholars, and Schizophrenics.* Berkeley: University of California Press.

Scull, Andrew (1979) *Museums of Madness.* New York: St Martin's Press.

Scull, Andrew (1984) *Decarceration: Community Treatment and the Deviant: A Radical View.* Rutgers, NJ: Rutgers University Press.

Scull, Andrew (ed.) (1981) *Madhouses, Mad-Doctors, and Madmen: The Social History of Psychiatry in the Victorian Era.* Philadelphia: University of Pennsylvania Press.

Skultans, Vieda (1975) *Madness and Morals: Ideas on Insanity in the Nineteenth Century.* London: Routledge.

Skultans, Vieda (1979) *English Madness: Ideas on Insanity.* London: Routledge.

Special Report From the Inspectors of the Lunatics to the Chief Secretary on the Alleged Increasing Prevalence of Insanity in Ireland. (1894) Dublin: Alexander Thom.

Tantam, D. (1991) The anti-psychiatry movement, in: G. Berrios and H. Freeman (eds) *150 Years of British Psychiatry.* London: Gaskell

Tomes, Nancy (1984) *A Generous Confidence: Thomas Story Kirkbride and the Art of Asylum-keeping, 1840–1883.* Cambridge: Cambridge University Press.

Torrey, E.F., M. McGuire, A. O' Hare, D. Walsh, and M. Spellman (1984) Endemic psychosis in the West of Ireland, *American Journal of Psychiatry,* 141: 8: 966–70.

Tracy, Honor (1953) *Mind You! I've Said Nothing: Forays in the Irish Republic.* Washington, DC: Robert B Luce.

Walsh, Dermot (1968) Hospitalized psychiatric morbidity in the Republic of Ireland, *British Journal of Psychiatry* 114: 11–14.

Warner, Richard (1985) *Recovery From Schizophrenia: Psychiatry and Political Economy.* London: Routledge.

World Health Organisation (1973) *International Pilot Study of Schizophrenia.* Geneva.

Notes on Contributors

Tanya M. Cassidy recently completed her doctoral studies at the Department of Sociology, University of Chicago on the historical and cultural influences surrounding the ambiguity associated with drinking in Ireland. She is currently living and working as a sociologist in Maynooth, Co. Kildare, Ireland.

Anne Cleary is a lecturer in the Department of Sociology at University College Dublin. Her research and lecturing interests include health and gender. She is a member of the board of the Health Research Board.

Claire Collins is the Surveys Executive in the Survey Unit of the Economic and Social Research Institute and was the Research Officer on the Kilkenny Health Project.

Ricca Edmondson has a DPhil from the University of Oxford and has worked at the Max Planck Institute for Human Development, Berlin. She now lectures in the Department of Political Science and Sociology at University College Galway and is director of the Centre for Intercultural Studies there.

Andrew Finlay lectures in sociology at Trinity College, Dublin; Dorothy Whittington and Monica McWilliams are based at the University of Ulster; Nicola Shaw is a researcher at the Northern Health and Social Services Board (NI). All of the authors were associated with the Centre for Health and Social Research at the University of Ulster when the research was carried out.

Abbey Hyde has a background in nursing and sociology. She is currently a lecturer in the Department of Nursing Studies, University College Dublin, having previously lectured at the University of Edinburgh. Her research interests include the politics of reproduction, nursing practices in relation to older people and the initiation of smoking in adolescence.

Desmond McCluskey is a lecturer in the Department of Sociology at University College Dublin. His principal teaching and research interests are in the sociology of health and medicine, disability, education and symbolic inter-action. He is the author of *Health: People's Beliefs and Practices*, Dublin Stationery Office, 1989.

Orla McDonnell lectures in sociology at University College Cork. Her current research interests are in the sociology of the body, health and medicine and feminist studies. She is completing her doctoral thesis on the social construction of infertility and the debate on the implications of advances in NRT.

Brian Nolan is a research economist at the Economic and Social Research Institute, Dublin (ESRI). He is joint editor of *Poverty and Policy in Ireland*, Gill & Macmillan 1994, and joint author of *Resources, Deprivation and Poverty*, Clarendon 1996, and *Poverty in the 1990s*, Oak Tree Press 1996. He has contributed papers on inequality, poverty and health to a range of international journals.

Orla O'Donovan is a lecturer in the Department of Applied Social Studies in University College Cork. Her research interests include health inequalities, Irish health policy and women's collective action.

Sam Porter trained as a general nurse at Coventry and subsequently returned to Ireland to take up a staff post at Whiteabbey Hospital. In 1987 he left to study sociology at Queen's University, Belfast, and has never escaped. He is now a lecturer in sociology at the University, specialising in the sociology of nursing.

A. Jamie Saris lectures in the Department of Anthropology, National University of Ireland, Maynooth. One of his research interests is how a large mental hospital in the west of Ireland effected certain historical changes at a particular locality and how it was, in turn, partially domesticated by local forces.

Emer Shelley is a public health specialist in the Eastern Health Board and was project leader on the Kilkenny Health Project.

Margaret P. Treacy is a nurse and sociologist and is head of the Department of Nursing Studies in University College Dublin. Her areas of interest include qualitative research, professional socialisation and health promotion.

Vincent Tucker was a lecturer in the Department of Sociology at University College Cork. His recent research focused on the sociology of health and the sociology of development. Vincent Tucker died in a road accident in March 1997.

Christopher T. Whelan is a research sociologist at ESRI. He is joint author of *Resources, Deprivation and Poverty*, Clarendon 1996, and *Poverty in the 1990s*, Oak Tree Press 1996. He has contributed papers on labour market marginalisation, psychological distress and the issue of an emerging underclass to a range of international journals.

Index